Ambulatory Care Nursing Exam Study Guide 2024-2025

Pass the ANCC Certification with Confidence: Detailed Content Review, Test-Taking Strategies, Full-Length Practice Tests and Detailed Answer Explanations

Test Treasure Publication

COPYRIGHT

All content, materials, and publications available on this website and through Test Treasure Publication's products, including but not limited to, study guides, flashcards, online materials, videos, graphics, logos, and text, are the property of Test Treasure Publication and are protected by United States and international copyright laws.

Copyright © 2024-2025 Test Treasure Publication. All rights reserved.

No part of these publications may be reproduced, distributed, or transmitted in any form or by any means, including photocopying, recording, or other electronic or mechanical methods, without the prior written permission of the publisher, except in the case of brief quotations embodied in critical reviews and certain other noncommercial uses permitted by copyright law.

Permissions

For permission requests, please write to the publisher, addressed "Attention: Permissions Coordinator," at the address below:

Test Treasure Publication

Email: support@testtreasure.com

Website: www.testtreasure.com

Unauthorized use or duplication of this material without express and written permission from this site's owner and/or author is strictly prohibited. Excerpts and links may be used, provided that full and clear credit is given to Test Treasure Publication with appropriate and specific direction to the original content.

Trademarks

All trademarks, service marks, and trade names used within this website and Test Treasure Publication's products are proprietary to Test Treasure Publication or other respective owners that have granted Test Treasure Publication the right and license to use such intellectual property.

Disclaimer

While every effort has been made to ensure the accuracy and completeness of the information contained in our products, Test Treasure Publication assumes no responsibility for errors, omissions, or contradictory interpretation of the subject matter herein. All information is provided "as is" without warranty of any kind.

Governing Law

This website is controlled by Test Treasure Publication from our offices located in the state of California, USA. It can be accessed by most countries around the world. As each country has laws that may differ from those of California, by accessing our website, you agree that the statutes and laws of California, without regard to the conflict of laws and the United Nations Convention on the International Sales of Goods, will apply to all matters relating to the use of this website and the purchase of any products or services through this site.

CONTENTS

Introduction	1
Brief Overview of the Ambulatory Care Nursing Exam and Its Importance	4
Detailed Content Review	8
Study Schedules and Planning Advice	16
Frequently Asked Questions	20
1. The Art of Ambulatory Care Nursing	26
2. The Art of Effective Communication	37
3. Navigating Professional Issues in Ambulatory Care Nursing	49
4. Mastering Information Literacy in Ambulatory Care	62
5. Advancing Education in Ambulatory Care	75
6.1 Full-Length Practice Test 1	92
6.2 Answer Sheet - Practice Test 1	120
7.1 Full-Length Practice Test 2	134
7.2 Answer Sheet - Practice Test 2	161
Test-Taking Strategies	175
Additional Resources	181
Final Words	188

Explore Our Range of Study Guides

INTRODUCTION

Welcome to the **"Ambulatory Care Nursing Exam Study Guide 2024-2025"**, a meticulously crafted resource designed to help you excel in your journey toward becoming a certified ambulatory care nurse. This study guide is not just another textbook—it's your personal companion, providing all the tools and knowledge you need to confidently approach the **Ambulatory Care Nursing Exam** and achieve success.

What is Ambulatory Care Nursing?

Ambulatory care nursing is a dynamic and essential branch of healthcare focused on delivering care to patients in outpatient settings. As an ambulatory care nurse, your role spans multiple responsibilities, including patient education, care coordination, health promotion, and disease management. With the growing demand for skilled nurses in this field, obtaining certification demonstrates your expertise and commitment to excellence.

Purpose of This Study Guide

This study guide has been tailored to align with the latest exam blueprint, covering all critical topics while ensuring a comprehensive and user-friendly approach. Whether you're just beginning your preparation or looking for a final review, this guide is structured to meet your needs and optimize your study experience.

What You'll Find in This Book

- **Exam Overview:** Understand the structure, administered body, significance, and expectations of the **Ambulatory Care Nursing Exam 2024-2025**.

- **In-Depth Content Review:** Covers essential topics, including **clinical practice, communication, professional issues, systems, and education**.

- **Practice Tests:** Two full-length practice exams with 100 questions each, complete with detailed answer explanations to strengthen your test-taking skills.

- **Test-Taking Strategies:** Proven methods to manage time, reduce anxiety, and maximize your performance on exam day.

- **Additional Resources:** Includes recommendations for further online and academic study materials.

- **Motivational Words:** Empowering messages to keep you focused and motivated throughout your preparation journey.

Who is This Guide For?

This book is perfect for:

- **Aspiring Ambulatory Care Nurses** preparing for certification.

- **Current Healthcare Professionals** seeking to expand their knowledge and skills.

- **Students and Educators** looking for comprehensive and reliable study material tailored to the latest standards.

How to Use This Guide

1. **Start with the Overview:** Familiarize yourself with the exam structure and key topics.

2. **Dive Into the Content:** Study each section carefully, using the provided examples, tips, and explanations.

3. **Practice, Practice, Practice:** Test your knowledge with the included practice tests and analyze your results to identify areas for improvement.

4. **Plan Your Study:** Use the recommended study schedules to stay organized and on track.

5. **Keep Going:** Stay motivated with practical advice and encouragement to help you achieve your goals.

Your Journey Starts Here

Certification as an ambulatory care nurse is a milestone that reflects your expertise, dedication, and professionalism. This study guide is your trusted resource, designed to simplify the preparation process and ensure your success. Together, let's take the first step toward achieving your dreams and advancing your career.

Welcome to a brighter future—let's get started!

Brief Overview of the Ambulatory Care Nursing Exam and Its Importance

The **Ambulatory Care Nursing Exam** is a nationally recognized certification test designed to validate your expertise and knowledge in the field of ambulatory care nursing. This certification demonstrates your commitment to excellence and positions you as a highly skilled professional in outpatient care settings. Administered by the **American Nurses Credentialing Center (ANCC)**, this exam is an essential step for advancing your career and staying competitive in today's healthcare industry.

Exam Details

Administered By:

- The **American Nurses Credentialing Center (ANCC)**, a globally respected organization that certifies nurses in various specialties.

Exam Format and Pattern:

- The **Ambulatory Care Nursing Exam** is a computer-based test (CBT) featuring multiple-choice questions. It is designed to assess your competency in delivering high-quality care in ambulatory settings.

Component	Details
Number of Questions	150 questions (125 scored and 25 pretest questions)
Type of Questions	Multiple-choice format
Exam Duration	3 hours
Question Topics	Clinical Practice, Communication, Professional Issues, Systems, and Education

Scoring:

- The test is scored on a **scale of 200 to 500**, with a minimum passing score of **350**. The scoring ensures an accurate evaluation of your proficiency in all key areas.

Eligibility Criteria:

- Active **RN license**.

- A minimum of **2 years' experience** as a registered nurse.

- At least **2,000 hours of clinical practice** in ambulatory care within the past 3 years.

- Completion of **30 hours of continuing education** in ambulatory care within the last 3 years.

Cost:

- ANCC Member: **$295**

- Non-Member: **$395**

Testing Locations:

- The exam is available at **Prometric testing centers** across the United States and online through remote proctoring.

Importance of the Exam

1. Professional Recognition:

Certification sets you apart as a highly competent professional and reinforces your expertise in ambulatory care nursing.

2. Career Advancement:

Certified nurses often qualify for leadership roles, higher salaries, and greater job opportunities.

3. Quality of Patient Care:

Certification demonstrates your dedication to providing evidence-based, patient-centered care in outpatient settings, ensuring improved patient outcomes.

4. Personal Fulfillment:

Achieving certification is a rewarding milestone that reflects your hard work, knowledge, and commitment to excellence in nursing.

5. Staying Competitive:

As ambulatory care evolves, certification ensures you remain knowledgeable about the latest practices and trends in the field.

This exam is a pivotal step in solidifying your role as an expert in ambulatory care nursing. With the knowledge, skills, and confidence gained from this study guide, you'll be fully equipped to succeed on the exam and excel in your nursing career. Let's move forward toward certification success!

DETAILED CONTENT REVIEW

The **"Ambulatory Care Nursing Exam Study Guide 2024-2025"** offers a comprehensive content review that aligns with the exam blueprint, covering all critical areas required for success. This section provides an in-depth exploration of the five primary content domains: Clinical Practice, Communication, Professional Issues, Systems, and Education.

1. The Clinical Practice

This section focuses on the core competencies required to deliver high-quality ambulatory care.

Key Topics:

- **Focal Points:**
  Understand essential nursing roles, including assessment, planning, implementation, and evaluation of patient care in outpatient settings.

    - Prioritization of patient care.

    - Integration of evidence-based practices.

- **Patient Advocate:**
  Explore the nurse's role as a patient advocate, ensuring patient rights, promoting autonomy, and addressing barriers to care.

- Navigating healthcare systems for patients.
- Advocating for equitable access to care.

- **Proper Triage:**
Learn effective triage strategies to prioritize care based on the severity of patient conditions.
    - Identifying urgent vs. non-urgent cases.
    - Utilizing standardized triage protocols.

- **Qualifications:**
Understand the qualifications and certifications that enhance the ambulatory care nurse's professional role.
    - Importance of continuing education.
    - Specialized certifications such as ANCC Ambulatory Care Nursing.

- **Care Management:**
Review strategies for coordinating care, managing chronic conditions, and implementing patient-centered care plans.
    - Interdisciplinary collaboration.
    - Transition and follow-up care.

2. The Communication

Communication is a cornerstone of effective nursing care, especially in outpatient settings.

Key Topics:

- **Telehealth Nursing Skills:**
  Learn to navigate virtual care environments and deliver high-quality telehealth services.

  - Building rapport remotely.

  - Managing technology challenges.

- **Documentation:**
  Master best practices in documentation to ensure legal compliance and support continuity of care.

  - Accurate recording of patient interactions.

  - Utilizing electronic health records (EHRs).

- **Cultural Competence:**
  Develop skills to provide culturally sensitive care and address diverse patient needs.

  - Understanding cultural values and beliefs.

  - Adapting communication styles.

- **Service Recovery Process:**
  Learn techniques for addressing patient complaints and improving satisfaction.

  - De-escalation strategies.

  - Building trust through resolution.

- **Informed Consent:**

Understand the nurse's role in obtaining and verifying informed consent.

- Explaining procedures and risks.
- Ensuring patient comprehension.

3. The Professional Issues

This section delves into legal, ethical, and leadership considerations critical to nursing practice.

Key Topics:

- **Licensure Issues:**
  Stay informed about licensure requirements and renewal processes.
  - Meeting continuing education criteria.
  - Avoiding common licensure pitfalls.

- **Incompetency and Informed Consent:**
  Address situations where patients may lack the capacity to provide informed consent.
  - Involving legal representatives.
  - Ethical considerations in care delivery.

- **Legal and Ethical Issues:**
  Explore the ethical principles that guide nursing practice and the legal responsibilities of nurses.

- Confidentiality and HIPAA compliance.
- Reporting unsafe practices.

- **Skills and Knowledge:**
Understand the key skills and knowledge areas for ambulatory care nurses.

    - Medication management.
    - Chronic disease education.

- **Leadership and Management:**
Learn to lead effectively within healthcare teams and manage resources efficiently.

    - Conflict resolution strategies.
    - Promoting a positive team culture.

4. The Systems

This section examines the operational and systemic aspects of ambulatory care nursing.

Key Topics:

- **Scheduling Patients:**
Review techniques for optimizing patient scheduling and reducing wait times.

    - Use of electronic scheduling systems.

- Managing high patient volumes.

- **Environmental Safety Issues:**
Understand safety protocols to maintain a secure care environment.

    - Identifying and mitigating hazards.

    - Conducting regular safety audits.

- **Conflict Resolution:**
Learn to resolve conflicts within healthcare teams and patient interactions effectively.

    - Communication strategies.

    - Mediation techniques.

- **Delegation of Duties:**
Master the art of delegation while ensuring compliance with scope of practice regulations.

    - Assigning tasks based on qualifications.

    - Monitoring outcomes.

- **Managed Care Plans:**
Explore the role of managed care in outpatient settings.

    - Coordinating patient care within cost-effective frameworks.

    - Understanding insurance requirements.

5. The Education

Education plays a vital role in empowering patients and promoting health.

Key Topics:

- **Health Promotion and Health Education:**
  Develop skills to educate patients about preventative measures and healthy lifestyle choices.
    - Smoking cessation programs.
    - Dietary and exercise recommendations.

- **Social Cognitive Theory:**
  Understand how this theory applies to nursing education and behavior change.
    - Building patient self-efficacy.
    - Reinforcement techniques.

- **Community Health:**
  Explore strategies to address public health challenges in outpatient care.
    - Partnering with local organizations.
    - Improving health equity.

- **Cultural Diversity:**
  Learn to deliver education tailored to diverse patient populations.
    - Respecting cultural beliefs in health education.
    - Overcoming language barriers.

- **Primary, Secondary, and Tertiary Health Prevention:**
  Review the nurse's role in all stages of health prevention.

    - Administering immunizations (primary).

    - Conducting screenings (secondary).

    - Managing rehabilitation programs (tertiary).

Additional Features

- **Tables and Charts:** Concise summaries of complex topics.

- **Tips and Tricks:** Practical advice for mastering difficult concepts.

- **Real-Life Scenarios:** Examples to enhance understanding and application.

This detailed content review ensures you have a comprehensive understanding of all exam topics. Use this guide to strengthen your knowledge, refine your skills, and approach the Ambulatory Care Nursing Exam with confidence!

Study Schedules and Planning Advice

Preparing for the **Ambulatory Care Nursing Exam** requires a strategic approach to ensure you cover all critical topics while managing your time effectively. This section provides study schedules and practical planning advice to help you stay on track and maximize your success.

How to Plan Your Study

Step 1: Assess Your Timeline

- Determine how much time you have before the exam date.
- Decide how many hours per day or week you can dedicate to studying.

Step 2: Understand the Exam Blueprint

- Familiarize yourself with the exam structure and focus on high-priority topics such as **clinical practice**, **communication**, **professional issues**, **systems**, and **education**.

Step 3: Set Goals

- Break down your study plan into manageable goals. Focus on one topic or sub-topic at a time to avoid overwhelm.

- Set weekly milestones to track your progress.

Step 4: Use Study Tools

- Utilize the resources provided in this guide, such as **content reviews**, **practice tests**, and **study tips**.

- Take advantage of additional online resources and reference materials.

Sample Study Schedules

Below are study schedules based on different preparation timelines. Adjust the schedule to fit your availability and learning style.

Week	Topics to Cover	Tasks
Week 1	Exam Overview & Clinical Practice	Review exam details, start with focal points, patient advocacy, triage, qualifications.
Week 2	Clinical Practice Continued	Focus on care management and practice related questions.
Week 3	Communication	Study telehealth skills, documentation, cultural competence, and informed consent.
Week 4	Professional Issues	Cover licensure, legal/ethical issues, and leadership skills.
Week 5	Systems	Study patient scheduling, safety, conflict resolution, delegation, and managed care plans.
Week 6	Education	Cover health promotion, social cognitive theory, cultural diversity, and prevention.
Week 7	Practice Tests	Take the first practice test and review explanations.
Week 8	Final Review	Focus on weak areas, review notes, and take the second practice test.

2. 4-Week Study Plan (Accelerated Preparation)

Week	Topics to Cover	Tasks
Week 1	Exam Overview, Clinical Practice & Communication	Review exam details, cover clinical practice, and start communication topics.
Week 2	Professional Issues & Systems	Focus on professional issues and systems topics, emphasizing key details.
Week 3	Education & Practice Test 1	Study education topics and take the first practice test.
Week 4	Review & Practice Test 2	Review weak areas, revise notes, and complete the second practice test.

3. 12-Week Study Plan (For Comprehensive Preparation)

Week	Topics to Cover	Tasks
Weeks 1-2	Exam Overview & Clinical Practice	Review exam details and cover clinical practice in detail.
Weeks 3-4	Communication	Study communication topics thoroughly and take notes.
Weeks 5-6	Professional Issues	Focus on legal/ethical issues, skills, and leadership topics.
Weeks 7-8	Systems	Study operational aspects like scheduling, safety, and conflict resolution.
Weeks 9-10	Education	Cover all education topics, including health promotion and prevention strategies.
Week 11	Practice Test 1 & Weak Areas	Take the first practice test, identify weaknesses, and revisit challenging topics.
Week 12	Final Review & Practice Test 2	Conduct a final review, take the second practice test, and focus on last-minute prep.

Tips for Successful Study Planning

1. **Create a Study Space:**

    Dedicate a quiet, distraction-free space for studying. Keep all your materials organized and accessible.

2. **Follow a Routine:**

    Consistency is key. Stick to a regular study schedule to establish a habit.

3. **Use Active Learning Techniques:**
   Engage with the material by summarizing, teaching others, or practicing questions instead of passive reading.

4. **Take Regular Breaks:**
   Follow the **Pomodoro Technique**: study for 25 minutes, then take a 5-minute break. This boosts focus and retention.

5. **Test Yourself Frequently:**
   Use the included practice tests and quiz yourself regularly to track progress and identify weak areas.

6. **Stay Healthy:**
   Prioritize self-care by eating well, staying hydrated, exercising, and getting enough sleep. A healthy mind is essential for effective studying.

7. **Seek Support:**
   Join online forums or study groups to share insights and motivation with peers.

Final Thoughts

Studying for the **Ambulatory Care Nursing Exam** can feel overwhelming, but with a well-structured plan and consistent effort, you can succeed. Use this guide to stay organized, track your progress, and focus on areas that need improvement. Remember, preparation is the key to confidence and success on exam day. Let's get started!

Frequently Asked Questions

1. What is the Ambulatory Care Nursing Exam?

The **Ambulatory Care Nursing Exam** is a certification test administered by the **American Nurses Credentialing Center (ANCC)**. It is designed to validate the knowledge, skills, and competencies of registered nurses working in outpatient care settings. Passing this exam earns you the **Ambulatory Care Nurse (AMB-BC)** credential, showcasing your expertise in this specialized field.

2. Why should I become certified in Ambulatory Care Nursing?

Certification demonstrates your commitment to professional development and excellence in ambulatory care. It enhances your credibility, opens doors to career advancement opportunities, and equips you with advanced knowledge to provide top-notch patient care. Certified nurses are often considered for leadership roles and enjoy increased job security.

3. What topics are covered on the exam?

The exam covers five major content areas:

- **Clinical Practice:** Patient care, advocacy, triage, and care management.
- **Communication:** Telehealth skills, documentation, cultural compe-

tence, and informed consent.

- **Professional Issues:** Licensure, ethical/legal considerations, and leadership.

- **Systems:** Scheduling, safety, conflict resolution, and managed care plans.

- **Education:** Health promotion, social cognitive theory, cultural diversity, and prevention strategies.

4. What is the format of the exam?

The exam consists of **150 multiple-choice questions**, of which **125 are scored** and **25 are pretest questions** (not scored). The test is computer-based and has a time limit of **3 hours**.

5. What is the passing score for the exam?

The exam is scored on a scale of **200 to 500**, with a passing score of **350**. Your score reflects your performance across all major content areas.

6. Am I eligible to take the exam?

To be eligible, you must meet the following criteria:

- Hold an **active RN license**.

- Have **2 years of experience** as a registered nurse.

- Accumulate **2,000 hours of clinical practice** in ambulatory care within the past 3 years.

- Complete **30 hours of continuing education** in ambulatory care within the last 3 years.

7. How should I prepare for the Ambulatory Care Nursing Exam?

Effective preparation includes:

- Studying a comprehensive guide like this one.
- Reviewing the exam blueprint and focusing on key topics.
- Practicing with full-length tests to familiarize yourself with the format.
- Utilizing test-taking strategies to manage time and reduce anxiety.

This guide includes detailed content reviews, two practice tests, and proven strategies to help you succeed.

8. What resources are included in this study guide?

This guide offers:

- **In-depth content review** for all exam topics.
- **Two full-length practice tests** with 100 questions each and detailed answer explanations.
- **Study schedules and planning advice** to help you stay organized.
- **Test-taking tips** to improve confidence and performance.
- **Additional resources** for further study and references.

9. Can I use this guide if I have limited study time?

Absolutely! This guide includes tailored study schedules for different timelines, including 4-week, 8-week, and 12-week plans. Even with limited time, you can focus on high-priority topics and practice questions to maximize your preparation.

10. Where can I take the exam?

The exam is available at **Prometric testing centers** across the United States and can also be taken online via **remote proctoring**.

11. How much does the exam cost?

The fee for the Ambulatory Care Nursing Exam is:

- **$295** for ANCC members.
- **$395** for non-members.
- Additional discounts may apply for members of partner organizations.

12. Can I retake the exam if I don't pass on the first attempt?

Yes, you can retake the exam. However, there are specific waiting periods and additional fees for retesting. Check the ANCC website for details on their retake policy.

13. Is this guide suitable for experienced nurses and beginners?

Yes! Whether you are a seasoned nurse looking to validate your expertise or a beginner seeking to expand your knowledge, this guide is designed to cater to all levels of experience.

14. How do I access the practice tests in this guide?

The practice tests are included within this book as printable materials. Each test consists of 100 questions, complete with detailed explanations for every answer to help you identify and address weak areas.

15. What are some test-taking strategies included in this guide?

This guide provides strategies to:

- Manage your time effectively during the exam.
- Eliminate incorrect answers using logic and reasoning.
- Stay calm under pressure with relaxation techniques.
- Focus on high-yield topics to maximize your score.

16. How long should I study before taking the exam?

This depends on your familiarity with the material and your available time. On average, candidates spend **6-12 weeks** preparing. The guide includes study schedules tailored for 4-week, 8-week, and 12-week preparation timelines.

17. Does this guide include online resources?

Yes, this guide recommends additional online resources and academic materials to complement your study plan and provide further insights into key topics.

18. What is the best way to use this guide?

Follow these steps:

1. **Start with the exam overview** to understand the structure and content.

2. **Study each section thoroughly**, using the summaries and tips.

3. **Take the practice tests** to assess your knowledge and improve weak areas.

4. **Review key topics** during the final weeks leading to the exam.

19. Can I use this guide as a reference after certification?

Absolutely! This guide can serve as a valuable resource for day-to-day nursing practice in ambulatory care settings.

20. Where can I find support if I have questions about the exam or this guide?

Feel free to reach out via the contact information provided in this guide or consult the ANCC website for detailed exam policies and updates.

1

THE ART OF AMBULATORY CARE NURSING

The Role of the Patient Advocate

A gentle breeze danced through the open window, carrying the scent of freshly bloomed flowers into the cozy examination room. The soft hum of the medical equipment provided a soothing backdrop as the nurse, Emma, sat beside her patient, Mrs. Wilson, a kind-faced elderly woman with a warm smile.

Emma's gentle demeanor and attentive presence immediately put Mrs. Wilson at ease. As they discussed her upcoming treatment plan, Emma listened intently, occasionally jotting down notes and asking thoughtful questions to ensure she fully understood Mrs. Wilson's concerns and preferences.

"I want you to know, Mrs. Wilson, that I'm here to advocate for you every step of the way," Emma said, her voice laced with compassion. "My role is to be your partner in this journey, to make sure your voice is heard and your needs are met."

Mrs. Wilson's eyes brightened, and she reached out to squeeze Emma's hand. "I'm so grateful to have you by my side, dear. This all feels a bit overwhelming, but knowing I have you to rely on makes me feel so much more at ease."

Emma smiled warmly, her gentle touch and soothing presence a testament to the crucial role of the patient advocate in ambulatory care settings. In these outpatient environments, where patients often navigate complex healthcare systems with limited support, the nurse's ability to effectively communicate, build trust, and empower patients is paramount.

As Mrs. Wilson shared her concerns about the upcoming treatment, Emma listened intently, nodding in understanding and offering reassuring words. "I know this can be a lot to take in, but I promise I'll be here to explain everything in a way that makes sense to you. Together, we'll make sure you have all the information you need to make the best decision for your health."

Emma's words were laced with a genuine concern and a deep understanding of the emotional and practical challenges facing her patient. She knew that navigating the healthcare system could be daunting, especially for the elderly or those with complex medical needs. That's why she made it her mission to be a trusted ally, guiding her patients through the process with patience, empathy, and unwavering support.

With a calm and nurturing demeanor, Emma gently walked Mrs. Wilson through the treatment options, explaining the potential benefits and risks in a way that was easy to understand. She encouraged Mrs. Wilson to ask questions, never shying away from difficult topics or technical jargon. In doing so, she empowered her patient to make an informed decision that aligned with her own values and preferences.

As the conversation drew to a close, Mrs. Wilson felt a sense of relief and confidence that she had not experienced in previous medical encounters. "I feel so much better about this now, Emma. You've really helped me understand what to expect, and I know I can count on you to be there for me."

Emma beamed with pride, knowing that her role as a patient advocate had made a meaningful difference in Mrs. Wilson's life. "I'll be with you every step of the way, Mrs. Wilson. You can count on that. I'm here to support you, to speak up for you, and to ensure your needs are always the top priority."

As Mrs. Wilson left the examination room, a renewed sense of hope and trust in the healthcare system filled her heart. The gentle, yet unwavering, presence of her patient advocate had made all the difference, reminding her that she was not alone in her journey to wellness.

Mastering Proper Triage

In the quiet of the ambulatory care clinic, the gentle hum of activity provided a soothing backdrop as the nurses and staff tended to the steady stream of patients. Among them, a young woman named Emily sat patiently, her eyes scanning the room with a hint of uncertainty. She had come in with a nagging cough, unsure of what to expect, but hoping the professionals here could provide the care and guidance she needed.

As Emily's name was called, she made her way to the triage station, where a warm-eyed nurse greeted her with a gentle smile. "How are you feeling today, Emily?" the nurse asked, her voice calming and reassuring.

"I've had this cough for a few days, and it just doesn't seem to be getting any better," Emily replied, her brow furrowed with concern. "I'm not sure what's causing it, and I'm a little worried."

The nurse nodded thoughtfully, already beginning the process of assessing Emily's condition. With practiced hands, she took Emily's vital signs, carefully monitoring her temperature, heart rate, and breathing. As she worked, she maintained a steady, soothing dialogue, explaining each step and reassuring Emily that she was in good hands.

"Okay, Emily, it looks like you're running a bit of a fever, but your other vital signs are within normal range," the nurse said, her tone gentle and reassuring. "Let's take a closer look and see if we can get to the bottom of this cough."

The nurse continued her assessment, asking Emily a series of targeted questions about her symptoms, medical history, and any potential triggers or exposures. With each query, she listened intently, her eyes filled with empathy and understanding.

As the examination progressed, the nurse's demeanor remained calm and composed, even as she delved into more complex aspects of Emily's condition. She explained the triage process in simple, easy-to-understand terms, guiding Emily through the steps with a steady hand and a comforting presence.

"Based on what we've seen so far, it looks like you may have a mild case of the flu," the nurse said, her voice laced with a hint of relief. "But don't worry, we have some great protocols in place to help get you back on your feet."

The nurse then outlined the appropriate course of treatment, outlining the evidence-based guidelines that would guide her care. She explained the rationale behind each recommendation, ensuring that Emily felt informed and empowered throughout the process.

As the nurse prepared the necessary medications and instructions, Emily couldn't help but feel a sense of reassurance wash over her. The nurse's attentive care and clear communication had allayed her initial concerns, and she now felt confident in the plan of action.

"Thank you so much for your help," Emily said, her voice tinged with gratitude. "I really appreciate how you've taken the time to explain everything to me."

The nurse smiled warmly, her gentle eyes conveying a genuine connection. "That's what we're here for, Emily," she replied. "Your health and well-being are our top priority. Now, let's get you started on that treatment plan and get you feeling better in no time."

As Emily made her way back to the waiting room, she couldn't help but feel a sense of comfort and security. The triage process had unfolded with a touch of whimsy and charm, the nurse's soothing language and soft, sensory imagery guiding her through the experience. Emily knew that she was in good hands, and she left the clinic feeling confident that her care would be both efficient and effective.

Qualifications for Ambulatory Care Nursing

Tucked away in the gentle folds of the healthcare landscape, the world of ambulatory care nursing beckons with a quiet allure. It is a realm where nurses, like quiet sentinels, guide patients through the intricate pathways of outpatient treatment, weaving a tapestry of compassion and expertise.

To don the mantle of an ambulatory care nurse is to embark on a journey of personal and professional growth, marked by a dedication to lifelong learning and a passion for providing personalized, holistic care. This subchapter delves into the qualifications and certifications that elevate the ambulatory care nurse, empowering them to navigate the nuances of this dynamic field with confidence and grace.

At the heart of ambulatory care nursing lies a deep understanding of the unique needs of patients who seek treatment outside the confines of the traditional hospital setting. These nurses must possess a keen eye for detail, a sharp clinical acumen, and the ability to adapt to the ever-evolving landscape of outpatient healthcare. Their role is not merely to administer treatment, but to cultivate a sense of trust and comfort, guiding patients through the complexities of their care with a gentle, reassuring touch.

The path to becoming an accomplished ambulatory care nurse begins with a solid foundation in nursing education. Aspiring nurses must first obtain a registered nursing (RN) license, which typically requires the completion of an accredited nursing program, whether it be a diploma, associate's, or bachelor's degree. This comprehensive training equips these caregivers with the fundamental knowledge and skills required to provide safe, effective, and holistic patient care.

However, the journey does not end there. Ambulatory care nursing demands a specialized set of competencies that go beyond the basic nursing curriculum. Nurses seeking to excel in this field must seek out additional educational opportunities, such as completing a post-graduate certificate program in ambulatory care nursing or pursuing a master's degree in nursing with a focus on outpatient care. These advanced programs delve into the intricacies of patient education, chronic disease management, care coordination, and the unique challenges that arise in the ambulatory care setting.

Alongside formal education, ambulatory care nurses must also stay attuned to the evolving best practices and emerging trends within their field. Continuous professional development, through workshops, conferences, and online learning modules, is essential to maintaining a sharp clinical edge and adapting to the ever-changing healthcare landscape. By embracing a spirit of lifelong learning, these nurses can ensure that their knowledge and skills remain current, allowing them to provide the highest quality of care to their patients.

To further solidify their expertise, many ambulatory care nurses pursue professional certifications, such as the Ambulatory Care Nursing Certification (ACNC) or the Certified Ambulatory Perioperative Nurse (CAPN) credential. These certifications demonstrate a nurse's comprehensive understanding of ambulatory care, and they are often viewed as a hallmark of excellence within the field. By attaining these credentials, nurses can not only enhance their own professional development but also contribute to the overall elevation of ambulatory care nursing as a specialized practice.

Beyond the academic and clinical qualifications, ambulatory care nurses must also possess a unique blend of personal attributes that complement their technical skills. Empathy, patience, and excellent communication skills are essential, as these nurses often engage in extensive patient education and collaborate closely with interdisciplinary teams. The ability to think critically, problem-solve, and adapt to changing circumstances is also crucial, as ambulatory care nurses must be prepared to navigate the dynamic and unpredictable nature of outpatient care.

Ultimately, the road to becoming an accomplished ambulatory care nurse is paved with a dedication to lifelong learning, a commitment to professional development, and a deep-rooted passion for providing exceptional patient-centered care. By embracing this multifaceted journey, nurses can unlock the true potential of ambulatory care, transforming the lives of patients one gentle, compassionate step at a time.

Care Management Strategies

As the sun peeked through the window, casting a warm glow across the cozy office, Nurse Emily settled into her chair, ready to embark on another day of caring for her patients. With a gentle smile, she began to reflect on the various strategies she employed in her ambulatory care nursing practice, each one a thread woven into the tapestry of holistic patient support.

Care Coordination: The Heart of the Matter

Emily's day often began with a careful review of her patient roster, mapping out the intricate web of their healthcare needs. Like a conductor orchestrating a symphony, she seamlessly coordinated the efforts of various healthcare providers, ensuring that each patient's care plan was a harmonious melody of specialized expertise. Whether arranging for a specialist consultation or facilitating the transfer of medical records, Emily's keen eye for detail and collaborative spirit were the driving forces behind her patients' seamless care experiences.

Guiding with a Nurturing Touch: Patient Education

As Emily greeted each patient, she made it a point to truly listen, to understand their unique concerns and goals. With a soothing tone and a nurturing touch, she would gently guide them through the complexities of their conditions, empowering them with the knowledge they needed to take an active role in their own well-being. Whether explaining the intricacies of a new medication or demonstrating the proper technique for managing a chronic illness, Emily's patience and personalized approach helped to allay their fears and foster a sense of confidence in their ability to navigate the healthcare landscape.

Unlocking the Pharmacy Puzzle: Medication Management

Medication management was a delicate dance in Emily's practice, requiring a meticulous eye and a deep understanding of each patient's unique needs. With a gentle touch, she would carefully review their medication regimens, ensuring that potential interactions were identified and addressed, and that dosages were tailored to their individual circumstances. Her role extended far beyond mere prescription refills; she became a trusted advisor, guiding her patients through the sometimes-bewildering world of pharmacology, offering insights and strategies to optimize their treatment outcomes.

Cultivating a Harmonious Collaboration: Interdisciplinary Teamwork

Emily's approach to patient care was not limited to her own expertise; rather, it was a symphony of collaborative efforts, harmonizing the specialized knowledge of various healthcare professionals. She seamlessly wove the insights of physicians, therapists, and other clinicians into a cohesive care plan, ensuring that each patient's needs were addressed from multiple angles. Through regular team meetings and open communication, Emily fostered a spirit of camaraderie and mutual respect, creating an environment where every member of the healthcare team felt valued and empowered to contribute to the patient's well-being.

A Tapestry of Compassion: Embracing the Whole Person

At the heart of Emily's care management strategies was a deep understanding that her patients were not merely a collection of symptoms or diagnoses, but whole individuals with unique stories, needs, and aspirations. She approached each encounter with a keen eye for the emotional and social factors that could impact their health, offering a listening ear and a gentle embrace when the burdens of illness threatened to become overwhelming. By weaving the threads of physical, mental, and emotional support into a tapestry of compassionate care, Emily ensured that her patients felt seen, heard, and cared for as unique human beings, not just patients.

As the sun began to dip below the horizon, Emily took a moment to reflect on the day's triumphs and challenges. Though the work was never truly done, she found solace in the knowledge that her dedication to holistic, patient-centered care had made a meaningful difference in the lives of those she served. With a renewed sense of purpose, she turned her gaze towards the future, eager to continue weaving the threads of her expertise, empathy, and unwavering commitment into the lives of her patients, one gentle gesture and thoughtful intervention at a time.

Anorexia Nervosa and Bulimia Nervosa in the Pediatric Population

The gentle patter of tiny feet echoes through the halls of the pediatric ward, a delicate symphony punctuated by the occasional soft giggle or sigh. Here, the challenges of caring for young patients with eating disorders like anorexia nervosa and bulimia nervosa take on a particularly poignant and sensitive nature.

With a touch of whimsy and a whisper of charm, the ambulatory care nurses navigate this terrain, offering a compassionate embrace to these fragile souls. Their role is not merely one of clinical expertise, but of nurturing guidance, a gentle hand to help these young individuals rediscover the joys of nourishing their bodies and minds.

As they approach each patient, the nurses are mindful of the delicate balance required – a dance of patience, understanding, and unwavering support. They know that these conditions, while often misunderstood, can cast a deep shadow over the vibrant spirits of their young charges, threatening to extinguish the very essence of childhood.

With a soft-spoken manner and a soothing touch, the nurses begin the assessment process, carefully weaving a tapestry of information that will guide the treatment plan. They rely on a variety of tools, each one designed to shed light on the unique challenges faced by these young patients, from standardized screening questionnaires to nuanced observations of behavior and emotional well-being.

The nurses understand that anorexia nervosa and bulimia nervosa are not just physical conditions, but deeply rooted in the complex interplay of psychological, social, and familial factors. They approach each case with a holistic perspective, recognizing that true healing requires addressing the mind, body, and spirit in equal measure.

As they collaborate with the multidisciplinary team of physicians, therapists, and nutritionists, the nurses become the conduit, translating the sometimes-daunting medical jargon into a language that the young patients and their families can understand. With empathy and patience, they guide them through the maze of treatment options, ensuring that each step is taken with the utmost care and consideration.

One of the most vital roles the nurses play is that of emotional support. They understand that the road to recovery is paved with challenges, both physical and emotional, and they are there to provide a steadfast shoulder to lean on. With a gentle touch and a soothing voice, they offer encouragement and reassurance, helping their young patients navigate the ups and downs of the healing process.

In the quiet moments, when the ward is bathed in the soft glow of night lamps, the nurses take time to listen to the whispered fears and dreams of their patients. They weave stories of hope and resilience, reminding these young individuals that they are not alone, that they are seen, and that they are worthy of healing and joy.

As the sun rises and the new day begins, the nurses are there, ready to face the challenges head-on. With a touch of whimsy and a spark of determination, they continue their mission, guiding these young souls towards a future where the beauty of childhood shines bright, unhindered by the shadows of eating disorders.

2

THE ART OF EFFECTIVE COMMUNICATION

Mastering Telehealth Nursing Skills

In the soft glow of the screen, the nurse's gentle voice guides her patient through a virtual consultation. With a touch of whimsy and a soothing cadence, she narrates the steps, creating a sense of comfort and ease in the digital realm. Though miles apart, the connection between them is palpable, a testament to the power of technology and the art of telehealth nursing.

Telehealth nursing has emerged as a transformative force in the healthcare landscape, blending the timeless wisdom of the nursing profession with the seamless integration of digital tools. It is a realm where technology and compassion coexist, where the barriers of distance melt away, and where patients can receive the care they need, all from the comfort of their own homes.

At the heart of this digital revolution lies the mastery of telehealth nursing skills – a tapestry of expertise woven with the threads of adaptability, empathy, and technological proficiency. It is a dance, of sorts, where the nurse gracefully navigates the virtual landscape, guiding patients through the intricate steps of remote monitoring, virtual consultations, and personalized education.

Let us embark on a journey through the enchanting world of telehealth nursing, where the senses are enveloped in a veil of gentle imagery and the rhythm of the interaction flows like a serene melody.

Remote Patient Monitoring: A Dance of Synchronicity

In the world of telehealth, remote patient monitoring is akin to a delicate waltz, where the nurse and the patient move in seamless synchronicity. Through the integration of cutting-edge devices and intuitive software, the nurse can closely track the vital signs, symptoms, and progress of their patients, all from the comfort of their own workspace.

Imagine a gentle breeze caressing the cheek of the patient as they effortlessly transmit their data, the technology acting as a conduit for their well-being. The nurse, with a keen eye and a discerning touch, reviews the information, weaving together the tapestry of the patient's health with each data point. It is a dance of vigilance and care, where the nurse's soothing presence is ever-present, even in the virtual realm.

Virtual Consultations: A Symphony of Compassion

When it comes to virtual consultations, the telehealth nurse becomes a maestro, orchestrating a symphony of compassion and clinical expertise. With a soft smile and a reassuring tone, they guide their patients through the digital landscape, ensuring that every interaction is infused with the warmth and personalization that has long been the hallmark of the nursing profession.

The virtual consultation unfolds like a well-choreographed performance, where the nurse's words and the patient's responses harmonize in perfect synergy. Through the use of cutting-edge video conferencing tools, the nurse can maintain eye contact, observe subtle cues, and engage in a meaningful dialogue, all while being physically distant.

It is a dance of trust and understanding, where the nurse's gentle presence and the patient's comfort become the melodies that weave the tapestry of a successful virtual consultation. With each interaction, the nurse adds a new layer of understanding, tailoring their approach to the unique needs and preferences of the individual, creating a truly personalized experience.

Patient Education: A Tapestry of Wellness

In the realm of telehealth nursing, patient education becomes a tapestry of wellness, woven with the threads of digital accessibility and personalized guidance. The nurse, armed with a wealth of knowledge and a passion for empowering their patients, becomes a beacon of health in the virtual world.

Imagine a nurse, their voice lilting with enthusiasm, guiding a patient through the intricacies of their condition, using interactive multimedia tools to bring the information to life. As the patient engages with the educational materials, they feel a sense of ownership over their health, like the author of their own wellness story.

The nurse, with a touch of whimsy and a keen understanding of the patient's needs, seamlessly integrates educational resources into the virtual consultation, creating a cohesive and enriching experience. From interactive videos to personalized care plans, the nurse weaves a tapestry of knowledge that empowers the patient to take an active role in their healthcare journey.

Challenges and Best Practices: Navigating the Digital Landscape

While the world of telehealth nursing is filled with enchantment and possibilities, it also presents unique challenges that require the nurse to be adaptable, resilient, and ever-vigilant. From ensuring the security and privacy of patient information to overcoming technological barriers, the telehealth nurse must possess a diverse skill set to navigate the digital landscape with grace and efficiency.

Yet, within these challenges lie the seeds of best practices – a garden of strategies that the telehealth nurse can cultivate to create a seamless and rewarding experience for both themselves and their patients. From establishing clear communication protocols to leveraging the power of virtual communities, the nurse becomes a guiding light, illuminating the path towards a future where telehealth nursing is the norm, rather than the exception.

In the end, the mastery of telehealth nursing skills is a journey of continuous learning and adaptation, where the nurse's unwavering commitment to patient-centered care becomes the driving force behind their success. It is a realm where technology and compassion converge, creating a symphony of healthcare that resonates with the rhythm of the modern world.

The Art of Documentation

In the tranquil world of ambulatory care nursing, where patients seek solace and healing, documentation holds a vital role – a delicate dance of precision, clarity, and the gentle embrace of the written word. Like a master weaver, the nurse must carefully craft a tapestry of patient records, each thread intricately woven to tell a story of care, progress, and the indelible connection between caregiver and those in their charge.

As the sun filters through the windows, casting a warm glow upon the serene clinic, the nurses set to their task with a sense of reverence. Their pens glide across the pages, capturing the nuances of each patient encounter with a touch of artistry. From the detailed history to the meticulous documentation of symptoms, vital signs, and treatment plans, the nurse's words become the threads that bind the patient's journey, preserving the delicate fabric of their care.

In this realm of ambulatory nursing, where the pace ebbs and flows like the gentle tide, the importance of accurate and comprehensive documentation cannot be overstated. It is the foundation upon which the entire healthcare team builds their understanding, collaborating seamlessly to ensure the best possible outcome for each individual entrusted to their care.

The nurse, with a keen eye and a steady hand, navigates the intricate web of documentation standards, ensuring that each entry adheres to the highest levels of precision and clarity. Like a virtuoso musician, they weave the nuances of the patient's story, capturing the subtle shifts in condition, the triumphs of recovery, and the delicate nuances that only a trained eye can discern.

As the day unfolds, the nurse's documentation becomes a tapestry of care, a testament to the diligence and attention to detail that defines the ambulatory nursing profession. Each entry, a brushstroke in the larger canvas of the patient's healthcare journey, serves as a vital link in the chain of communication, enabling seamless collaboration and informed decision-making by the entire healthcare team.

But the art of documentation extends beyond the mere recording of facts and figures. It is a delicate balance of legal considerations, safeguarding both the patient and the healthcare provider. The nurse, with a keen understanding of the legal landscape, ensures that every word, every detail, is documented with the utmost care, creating a comprehensive record that serves as a shield against potential challenges and a testament to the quality of care provided.

In the tranquil sanctuary of the ambulatory care clinic, the nurse's pen becomes a wand of empowerment, transforming the mundane into the extraordinary. Through their diligent and thoughtful documentation, they not only preserve the integrity of the patient's care but also empower their colleagues, equipping them with the information they need to provide the highest level of treatment and support.

As the sun dips below the horizon, casting a warm glow over the quieting clinic, the nurses pause, their work complete for the day. They take a moment to reflect on the tapestry they have woven, the stories they have preserved, and the lives they have touched through the art of documentation. For in this realm of ambulatory care, where the gentle rhythm of healing prevails, the nurse's words become the symphony that guides the patient's journey, a symphony of care, compassion, and the enduring power of the written record.

Cultural Competence in Ambulatory Care

In the gentle hush of the waiting room, the soothing chime of the receptionist's voice beckons patients to come forth, each with their own unique stories and cultural tapestries woven into the fabric of their lives. As the ambulatory care nurse, it is our sacred duty to navigate this tapestry with the utmost care and sensitivity, ensuring that every individual who crosses our threshold feels welcomed, understood, and empowered in their healthcare journey.

Cultural competence is the elegant dance between understanding and embracing the rich diversity that surrounds us. It is the gentle unfolding of curiosity, the willingness to learn, and the deep respect for the beliefs, practices, and experiences that shape each person's perspective on wellness and healing. Much like the delicate petals of a blooming flower, cultural competence blossoms when we approach our patients with an open heart, a curious mind, and a reverence for the myriad of ways in which they view the world.

As ambulatory care nurses, we bear witness to the intricate interplay between cultural beliefs and healthcare delivery. Whether it is the reverence for traditional herbal remedies or the significance of family involvement in the decision-making process, understanding these nuances is paramount to providing care that is truly responsive to the needs of our patients. By embracing this cultural tapestry, we can create a safe and inclusive environment where individuals feel empowered to share their stories, express their concerns, and actively participate in their own well-being.

Building cultural competence is a journey of continuous learning and self-reflection. It requires us to shed our preconceptions, to challenge our own biases, and to approach each encounter with a beginner's mind. Through open and honest dialogue, we can learn about the diverse perspectives and lived experiences that shape our patients' worldviews. By actively seeking to understand the cultural, spiritual, and social factors that influence their healthcare decisions, we can tailor our approach to address their unique needs and preferences.

In the realm of ambulatory care, the nurse plays a pivotal role in fostering cultural competence. We are the gentle guides, the attentive listeners, and the compassionate advocates who strive to bridge the gap between the healthcare system and the rich diversity of the communities we serve. With a keen eye for detail and a heart full of empathy, we can navigate the intricate landscape of cultural beliefs, customs, and communication styles, ensuring that every interaction is a meaningful and empowering experience.

From the moment a patient steps through the door, the nurse's role is to create a welcoming and inclusive environment. This may involve simple gestures, such as displaying culturally diverse artwork, providing translation services, or offering reading materials in multiple languages. By acknowledging and honoring the cultural identities of our patients, we communicate a powerful message of respect and understanding, setting the stage for a collaborative and trust-filled partnership.

As we delve deeper into the realm of cultural competence, we must also be mindful of the challenges and nuances that can arise. Language barriers, differing perceptions of time and personal space, and varying levels of health literacy can all present unique obstacles to effective communication and care coordination.

However, with a deep well of patience, flexibility, and a genuine desire to understand, we can navigate these challenges with grace and compassion.

In the end, the pursuit of cultural competence in ambulatory care is not merely a professional obligation, but a sacred calling. It is the gentle unfolding of understanding, the deliberate cultivation of empathy, and the unwavering commitment to providing care that honors the unique stories and perspectives of each individual who entrusts us with their well-being. By embracing this journey, we not only enhance the quality of care we deliver, but we also become the humble stewards of a more inclusive and equitable healthcare landscape, where every patient feels seen, heard, and empowered to thrive.

Mastering the Service Recovery Process

In the serene halls of an ambulatory care setting, where the air is laced with the gentle hum of medical equipment and the reassuring presence of compassionate caregivers, a delicate dance unfolds – the art of service recovery. This graceful choreography, woven with empathy and problem-solving, is the cornerstone of ensuring patient satisfaction and fostering a harmonious healthcare experience.

As patients navigate the sometimes-complex landscape of modern healthcare, they may encounter moments where their expectations are not fully met. It is in these instances that the service recovery process shines, a beacon of understanding and problem-solving that can transform a challenging situation into a resounding success.

At the heart of this process lies the power of communication – a delicate balance of active listening, genuine concern, and thoughtful responses. Imagine a patient, perhaps feeling frustrated or confused, approaching the care team with a concern. The skilled service recovery practitioner listens intently, their eyes reflecting the patient's emotions, their words carrying a soothing cadence that invites the patient to fully express their thoughts and feelings.

With a gentle touch and a calming presence, the practitioner acknowledges the patient's experiences, validating their concerns and demonstrating a genuine desire to understand. This empathetic approach creates an environment of trust, where the patient feels heard, respected, and empowered to work alongside the care team to find a solution.

The next step in this harmonious dance is the art of conflict resolution. In the face of a patient complaint or a challenging situation, the service recovery practitioner navigates with the grace of a skilled diplomat, deftly addressing the root of the issue and exploring mutually beneficial resolutions. Through open-ended questions and a collaborative spirit, they uncover the nuances of the problem, seeking to understand the patient's perspective and pinpoint the underlying causes.

With a keen eye for detail and a solutions-oriented mindset, the practitioner then skillfully crafts a response that not only addresses the immediate concern but also offers a path forward. This could involve adjusting processes, providing additional resources, or simply offering a sincere apology – all with the aim of restoring the patient's trust and leaving them feeling valued and cared for.

Mastering the service recovery process in the ambulatory care setting is akin to a delicate dance, where each step is choreographed with intention and grace. It is a dance of empathy, problem-solving, and a steadfast commitment to patient satisfaction. By embracing this art, healthcare providers can transform moments of potential disappointment into opportunities for deeper connection, enhanced trust, and a renewed sense of confidence in the care they provide.

As patients navigate the complexities of their healthcare journeys, the service recovery process becomes a guiding light, a beacon of hope that reminds them that their well-being is the top priority. Through this harmonious interplay of compassion and problem-solving, the ambulatory care setting becomes a sanctuary where patients can feel truly cared for, their concerns addressed with the utmost care and attention.

In the end, the service recovery process is not just a set of protocols or procedures – it is a testament to the fundamental values of healthcare, a reflection of the deep-rooted commitment to putting patients first and ensuring their needs are met with the utmost care and diligence. By mastering this art, healthcare providers can create an environment of trust, empowerment, and unwavering support, where patients feel truly seen, heard, and empowered to actively participate in their own healthcare journey.

Communicating With Non-English Speaking Patients

Stepping into the bright, airy clinic, Dr. Sophia Garcia greeted her next patient with a warm smile. As she approached the waiting area, she noticed a young woman, hands folded in her lap, gaze fixed on the floor. Sensing the woman's unease, Sophia approached her slowly, her steps gentle, her expression soothing.

"Good morning," Sophia said, her voice soft and melodic. The woman looked up, her eyes wide with uncertainty. "My name is Dr. Garcia. I'm here to help you today. I understand you may not speak much English. Please, don't worry - we have an interpreter who will be joining us shortly to assist with our visit."

The woman nodded, her shoulders relaxing ever so slightly. Sophia gestured for her to follow, guiding her to the examination room with a calm, unhurried pace. As they walked, Sophia took in the woman's appearance - the delicate floral scarf draped over her shoulders, the intricate embroidery on her sleeve. She made a mental note to be mindful of cultural differences and traditions, wanting to make the patient feel at ease.

Moments later, a gentle knock at the door signaled the arrival of the interpreter, a kind-faced woman named Maria. With a reassuring nod, Sophia introduced the two, explaining that Maria would be there to facilitate their conversation. The patient's eyes lit up with relief, and she immediately began speaking in her native tongue, her words flowing with a musical cadence.

Sophia listened intently, nodding along as Maria translated. She asked gentle, open-ended questions, allowing the patient to share her concerns at her own pace. When the woman hesitated, unsure of the right words, Maria offered thoughtful prompts, guiding the conversation with a deft touch.

As the visit progressed, Sophia took care to use simple, easily understood language, pausing frequently to ensure the patient fully grasped the information. She supplemented her explanations with hand gestures and diagrams, drawing on her years of experience in providing culturally sensitive care.

When it came time to discuss the treatment plan, Sophia made a concerted effort to involve the patient in the decision-making process. She explained the options in clear, straightforward terms, occasionally glancing at Maria to gauge the patient's level of understanding. With the interpreter's help, the woman asked thoughtful questions, her brow furrowed in concentration.

Sophia could sense the patient's growing comfort as the visit unfolded. The initial tension had given way to a sense of mutual trust and respect. She made a mental note to schedule a follow-up appointment, ensuring the patient had ample time to process the information and feel empowered in her own care.

As the patient prepared to leave, Sophia placed a gentle hand on her arm, her eyes shining with compassion. "I'm so glad we were able to connect today," she said, her words accompanied by a warm smile. "Please, don't hesitate to reach out if you have any other questions or concerns. We're here to support you every step of the way."

The patient nodded, her expression softening. With a heartfelt "thank you," she followed Maria out of the room, her steps more assured, her gaze filled with a newfound sense of understanding and reassurance.

Sophia watched them go, a quiet satisfaction blooming in her chest. Moments like these were a reminder of why she had chosen this path - to provide compassionate, culturally sensitive care, to bridge the gaps that so often arise between providers and patients. With a deep breath, she turned her attention to the next patient, ready to embark on another journey of mutual understanding and healing.

3

NAVIGATING PROFESSIONAL ISSUES IN AMBULATORY CARE NURSING

Licensure Issues in Ambulatory Care Nursing

As the sun rose gently over the bustling city, casting a warm glow across the bustling streets, Lily stepped out into the crisp morning air. The gentle hum of activity surrounded her as she made her way to the hospital, her nursing scrubs crisp and her step filled with purpose.

Lily was an ambulatory care nurse, a dedicated professional whose role was to provide compassionate, high-quality care to patients in outpatient settings. It was a calling that filled her with a deep sense of purpose, and she took great pride in the skills and knowledge she had honed over the years.

As she arrived at the hospital, Lily paused for a moment to take in the scene before her. The lobby was alive with activity, patients and their families bustling to and fro, each seeking the care and support they needed. Lily knew that her role was crucial in this bustling environment, and she was determined to ensure that every patient who walked through those doors received the best possible care.

One of the key aspects of Lily's work was the regulatory and licensure requirements that governed the field of ambulatory care nursing. In order to practice as a nurse in this specialized setting, Lily needed to maintain a valid nursing license, as well as any additional certifications or credentials that were required by her state or employer.

The process of obtaining and maintaining these professional credentials was not always simple, but Lily understood the importance of staying up-to-date and compliant. "It's not just about meeting the legal requirements," she said, her voice filled with a gentle determination. "It's about ensuring that I have the knowledge and skills to provide the best possible care to my patients. I take great pride in being a skilled and knowledgeable ambulatory care nurse, and I'm committed to continuing my professional development throughout my career."

Lily's commitment to her profession was evident in the way she approached her work. As she made her rounds, greeting patients with a warm smile and a gentle demeanor, she took the time to listen to their concerns and address their needs with the utmost care and attention. Whether it was administering medication, providing education on chronic conditions, or coordinating with other members of the healthcare team, Lily approached each task with the same level of dedication and expertise.

One of the unique challenges of ambulatory care nursing was the need to navigate the complex web of state-level regulations and licensure requirements. Each state had its own set of rules and regulations governing the practice of nursing, and it was crucial for Lily and her colleagues to stay informed and up-to-date on these ever-evolving guidelines.

Fortunately, Lily had a strong support system in place, both within her hospital and through professional organizations like the American Academy of Ambulatory Care Nursing (AAACN). These resources provided valuable information and guidance on the latest licensure requirements, as well as opportunities for professional development and networking.

As Lily made her way through the hospital, she couldn't help but reflect on the significance of her role. "Ambulatory care nursing is a unique and rewarding field," she said, her eyes shining with a sense of pride. "We get to be the first point of contact for so many patients, and we have the opportunity to truly make a difference in their lives. It's a responsibility that I take very seriously, and I'm honored to be a part of this incredible community of healthcare professionals."

With a renewed sense of purpose, Lily continued on her rounds, her steps filled with the gentle rhythm of her work. As she moved from one patient to the next, she knew that her commitment to excellence, her passion for her profession, and her dedication to maintaining the highest standards of licensure and certification were all integral to the care she provided. It was a responsibility she embraced with open arms, driven by a deep desire to make a positive impact on the lives of those she served.

Incompetency and Informed Consent

On a sun-dappled afternoon, Nurse Emma made her rounds through the quiet halls of the community clinic. As she moved from one patient room to the next, a gentle air of kindness and attentiveness surrounded her. Emma understood that each interaction was an opportunity to guide her patients with a steady hand, ensuring their wellbeing and empowering them to make informed decisions about their care.

One of Emma's patients that day was Mrs. Hollingsworth, a beloved member of the neighborhood who had been coming to the clinic for years. Now in her late 80s, Mrs. Hollingsworth's memory was starting to fail, and Emma could see the growing concern in the older woman's eyes. Sitting down beside her, Emma spoke softly, assessing Mrs. Hollingsworth's capacity to make decisions about her own healthcare.

"How are you feeling today, Mrs. Hollingsworth?" Emma asked, her voice soothing and patient.

The older woman paused, her brow furrowed in concentration. "I'm... I'm not quite sure, to be honest," she admitted, her words tentative. "I've been so forgetful lately, and the doctors keep telling me different things."

Emma nodded sympathetically, placing a gentle hand on Mrs. Hollingsworth's arm. "I understand this must be a difficult time for you. But I want you to know that I'm here to help guide you through it, every step of the way."

Carefully, Emma explained the concept of informed consent, emphasizing the importance of Mrs. Hollingsworth's autonomy in making decisions about her own care. She described the various treatment options, outlining the potential risks and benefits in a clear, accessible manner. Throughout the conversation, Emma kept a watchful eye, observing the older woman's responses and ensuring that she was fully engaged and comprehending the information.

Mrs. Hollingsworth listened intently, her eyes slowly regaining their familiar spark of understanding. "I think I'd like to try the new medication the doctor recommended," she said, her voice steady. "But I want to make sure I understand all the details before I sign anything."

Emma smiled warmly. "That's wonderful, Mrs. Hollingsworth. I'm so proud of you for taking the time to carefully consider your options. Let's go through the consent form together, and I'll make sure you have all the information you need to make the best decision for your health."

As the afternoon wore on, Emma encountered similar situations with other patients, each one unique in their own way. Some struggled with cognitive impairments, while others faced language barriers or emotional challenges. But Emma's approach remained steadfast – empathetic, patient, and focused on preserving her patients' autonomy and right to self-determination.

In one particularly poignant encounter, Emma met with a young man named Aiden, who had recently been diagnosed with a chronic condition. Aiden was visibly anxious, unsure of what the future held and overwhelmed by the barrage of medical information he'd received.

"I just feel so lost," Aiden confessed, his hands trembling. "The doctors keep talking about all these treatments, but I don't know what to choose. I'm scared I'm going to make the wrong decision."

Emma listened intently, her eyes filled with compassion. "I know this is a lot to take in, Aiden," she said, her voice soothing. "But I want you to know that you're not alone. Together, we're going to make sure you have all the information you need to make the best decision for your health and well-being."

Carefully, Emma walked Aiden through the treatment options, answering his questions and addressing his concerns. She encouraged him to take his time, to weigh the pros and cons, and to trust his instincts. As Aiden slowly regained his composure, Emma could see the spark of determination returning to his eyes.

"I think I'd like to try the medication," Aiden said, his voice steadier. "But I want to make sure I understand all the risks and side effects before I sign anything."

Emma nodded approvingly. "That's a wise decision, Aiden. Let's go through the consent form together, and I'll make sure you have all the details you need to feel confident in your choice."

As the sun began to set, casting a warm glow over the clinic, Emma reflected on the day's encounters. Each patient had presented unique challenges, but through it all, she had remained steadfast in her commitment to preserving their autonomy and empowering them to make informed decisions. It was a delicate balance, requiring a deep understanding of both the legal and ethical considerations surrounding competency and consent.

But for Emma, it was more than just a professional obligation – it was a calling, a way to make a meaningful difference in the lives of those she served. With each conversation, she strived to foster a sense of trust and understanding, guiding her patients through the complexities of the healthcare system with a gentle hand and a compassionate heart.

As she prepared to head home, Emma knew that tomorrow would bring new challenges, new faces, and new opportunities to make a difference. But she was ready, her dedication to her patients unwavering. For in the end, it was not the accolades or the awards that mattered most, but the knowledge that she had made a lasting impact on the lives of those she had been entrusted to care for.

Legal and Ethical Issues in Ambulatory Care

As the sun's gentle rays peeked through the windows of the cozy ambulatory care center, the nurses exchanged soft smiles, their steps light and purposeful. They knew that today, as every day, they would be navigating the delicate balance between providing exceptional care and honoring the legal and ethical principles that guided their work.

Confidentiality, the unspoken promise whispered between caregiver and patient, was the cornerstone of their practice. The nurses moved through the corridors, their voices hushed, their movements fluid, ever mindful of the sensitive information entrusted to them. They knew that each person who walked through the doors sought not only medical attention, but also the assurance that their most intimate details would be safeguarded with the utmost care.

Privacy, a cherished right in the world of healthcare, was woven into the very fabric of the center. The nurses carefully crafted a sanctuary where patients could feel at ease, unencumbered by the prying eyes of the outside world. They understood that in this serene space, individuals could open their hearts and minds, secure in the knowledge that their vulnerabilities would be treated with the utmost respect.

Liability, a word that carried weight, was not to be taken lightly. The nurses knew that their actions, their decisions, their very presence, could have profound consequences. They approached each encounter with a deep sense of responsibility, always mindful of the trust placed in their hands. Their training, their experience, and their unwavering dedication to the well-being of their patients, served as the foundation upon which they built their practice.

Ethical dilemmas, the subtle shades of gray that sometimes clouded the way forward, were navigated with a delicate touch. The nurses understood that their role extended far beyond the physical realm, encompassing the emotional, the spiritual, and the moral. They were not mere technicians, but healers, guides, and advocates, each decision informed by a steadfast commitment to the principles of beneficence, non-maleficence, autonomy, and justice.

As the day unfolded, the nurses deftly wove these complex threads together, creating a tapestry of care that was both reassuring and empowering. They listened with open hearts, offered guidance with a gentle touch, and upheld the inviolable trust that had been placed in them. In this sanctuary of healing, they found solace, purpose, and the unwavering knowledge that their work was not just a job, but a calling – a sacred responsibility to those who had entrusted their well-being to their capable hands.

Skills and Knowledge Development

As the sun gently peeked through the window, casting a warm glow over the cozy ambulatory care clinic, Lily took a moment to reflect on her journey as a nurse. The soft patter of rain against the glass reminded her of the ever-evolving nature of her profession, a constant reminder to embrace the pursuit of knowledge and growth.

Lily had always been a curious soul, eager to learn and explore the latest advancements in her field. She knew that in the ever-changing landscape of healthcare, staying up-to-date with the latest evidence-based practices was not just a professional obligation, but a personal passion. With a gentle smile, she settled into her chair, ready to dive into the world of continuing education opportunities that would shape her development as an ambulatory care nurse.

As she scrolled through the upcoming workshop listings, Lily's eyes lit up with excitement. From the latest advancements in chronic disease management to the cutting-edge techniques in patient-centered care, the options were endless. She carefully selected a few that piqued her interest, eager to immerse herself in the knowledge and insights that would help her better serve her patients.

Attending these workshops was more than just a chance to earn continuing education credits; it was an opportunity to connect with her peers, share experiences, and learn from the collective wisdom of the nursing community. Lily cherished these moments, where she could engage in thoughtful discussions, explore new perspectives, and gain a deeper understanding of the nuances that defined her role as an ambulatory care nurse.

But Lily's pursuit of knowledge didn't stop at the classroom doors. She found herself constantly seeking out the latest research, scouring medical journals and professional publications for the latest breakthroughs and innovations. With a keen eye and an insatiable curiosity, she meticulously analyzed the findings, eager to translate the evidence into tangible improvements in her own practice.

As she delved deeper into the world of research, Lily discovered that the journey of knowledge development was not just about acquiring information – it was about cultivating a critical mindset, one that challenged assumptions, questioned the status quo, and sought to push the boundaries of what was possible in patient care.

Guided by this spirit of inquiry, Lily found herself exploring new avenues of professional growth, from spearheading quality improvement initiatives to collaborating with interdisciplinary teams on innovative care models. Each step of the way, she embraced the opportunity to learn, to grow, and to make a meaningful impact on the lives of her patients.

In the quiet moments between patients, Lily would often pause and reflect on the transformative power of continuous learning. She knew that her role as an ambulatory care nurse was not just about delivering skilled medical care; it was about being a trusted partner, a compassionate advocate, and a lifelong learner, committed to delivering the highest quality of care.

With a deep breath, Lily turned her attention to the task at hand, her mind brimming with the knowledge and insights she had gained through her relentless pursuit of professional development. As she greeted her next patient, she carried with her a sense of purpose, a genuine desire to make a difference, and a steadfast commitment to the principles of evidence-based practice that had become the cornerstone of her nursing career.

Leadership and Management in Ambulatory Care

As the sun peeked through the windows of the bustling ambulatory care clinic, Nurse Emily took a deep breath and surveyed the day ahead. She knew that navigating the delicate balance of teamwork, conflict resolution, and quality improvement would require a deft touch – but she was up for the challenge.

Stepping into her office, Emily gazed upon the lush potted plants that lined the windowsill, a small touch of nature to soothe the hectic pace of the clinic. She settled into her chair, running a gentle hand across the smooth wood grain, and began to organize her thoughts.

As the leader of the nursing team, Emily understood the importance of fostering a collaborative environment. "It takes a village," she mused, her fingers tracing the outline of her favorite coffee mug. With a soft smile, she recalled the team-building exercises she had implemented, designed to nurture a sense of camaraderie and open communication.

From monthly team lunches to quarterly off-site retreats, Emily had woven little moments of connection into the fabric of their workdays. Whether it was sharing a laugh over a shared triumph or rallying around a difficult case, her nurses had developed a bond that transcended the typical work relationships.

Yet, Emily also knew that conflict was an inevitable part of any team dynamic. With a practiced hand, she had learned to navigate those treacherous waters, approaching each situation with a calm demeanor and an open mind. "Conflict can be a catalyst for growth," she murmured, "if we approach it with empathy and understanding."

Emily recalled a particularly delicate situation that had arisen the previous month. Two of her nurses, both passionate and dedicated, had found themselves at odds over the best course of treatment for a particularly complex patient. Rather than let the disagreement fester, Emily had gently intervened, guiding them through a thoughtful discussion and helping them reach a compromise that honored both of their perspectives.

In the end, the patient had benefited from the combined expertise of the nursing team, and the two nurses had emerged with a renewed respect for one another's skills and insights. Emily smiled, proud of the way her team had navigated the challenge, growing stronger in the process.

As the morning sun climbed higher in the sky, Emily turned her attention to the task of driving quality improvement throughout the clinic. She knew that complacency was the enemy of excellence, and she was determined to foster a culture of continuous learning and innovation.

With a gentle tap of her pen against the notepad, Emily began to outline her plans for the upcoming staff meeting. She would share the latest industry best practices, encourage her nurses to share their own ideas and insights, and together, they would identify areas for improvement.

Perhaps they could explore ways to streamline the patient intake process, or investigate new technologies that could enhance the patient experience. Emily's eyes gleamed with excitement at the prospect of empowering her team to make a tangible difference in the lives of their patients.

As the day wore on, Emily moved through the clinic, her presence a calming influence amidst the bustling activity. She paused to offer a word of encouragement to a nurse struggling with a particularly challenging case, and she made a mental note to check in with the newest member of the team, ensuring that she felt supported and valued.

In the quiet moments, Emily reflected on the privilege of her role as a leader in ambulatory care nursing. It was a delicate dance, balancing the needs of her team, the expectations of her patients, and the ever-evolving landscape of healthcare. But with her unwavering commitment to excellence and her deep well of empathy, Emily was more than up to the task.

As the sun began to dip below the horizon, Emily gathered her things and headed home, her mind already turning to the challenges and opportunities that the next day would bring. With a gentle smile and a renewed sense of purpose, she knew that she was exactly where she was meant to be, guiding her team and her patients towards a future filled with compassion, innovation, and the very best in ambulatory care.

The Impact of Social Networking

In the enchanting meadow of modern healthcare, the delicate dance between technology and patient care has become a symphony of endless possibilities. As the sun's gentle rays filter through the swaying branches, the impact of social networking on the realm of ambulatory nursing unfolds like a captivating melody.

Once upon a time, the nurse's domain was confined to the walls of the hospital, their reach limited by the confines of physical space. But just as the breeze carries the scent of wildflowers, the digital age has ushered in a new era, where the boundaries of care have become as boundless as the horizon.

Imagine a world where a nurse, with a few taps of their fingertips, can connect with a community of fellow practitioners, sharing insights, collaborating on projects, and harnessing the collective wisdom of the profession. This is the power of social networking, a tapestry woven with threads of collaboration, education, and camaraderie.

Through the vibrant channels of social media, ambulatory nurses can now forge connections that transcend geographical barriers, cultivating a thriving network of support and knowledge. It's as if a enchanted forest has sprung to life, where each tree represents a unique voice, a wellspring of experience, and a treasure trove of best practices.

But the true beauty of this digital landscape lies not just in the professional networking it enables, but in the way it empowers nurses to educate and empower their patients. Imagine a patient, anxious and uncertain, finding solace in the warm glow of their screen, where a nurse's soothing voice and carefully curated content gently guide them through the complexities of their healthcare journey.

With the touch of a button, nurses can share educational resources, offer personalized advice, and foster a sense of community that transcends the confines of the clinic. It's as if the nurse has become a trusted companion, walking alongside the patient every step of the way, even when physical distance separates them.

Yet, as with any enchanted forest, there are shadows that lurk, reminders of the ethical considerations that must be woven into the tapestry of social networking in healthcare. The delicate balance of privacy and confidentiality must be navigated with the utmost care, like a skilled dancer treading lightly on a moonlit path.

Nurses must tread carefully, mindful of the digital footprints they leave behind, ensuring that the trust placed in them by their patients is never betrayed. It's a dance of grace and discretion, where each step is choreographed with the utmost respect for the sanctity of patient information.

As the sun dips below the horizon, casting a warm glow over the meadow, one can't help but marvel at the transformative power of social networking in the realm of ambulatory nursing. It's a symphony of innovation and compassion, a harmonious blend of technology and the timeless art of healing.

And just as the stars begin to twinkle in the evening sky, a new chapter unfolds, where nurses and patients alike embark on a journey of discovery, where the boundaries of care are as limitless as the human spirit itself.

4

MASTERING INFORMATION LITERACY IN AMBULATORY CARE

Efficient Patient Scheduling

The hush of the waiting room was punctuated by the gentle chime of the receptionist's computer, as she effortlessly navigated the patient scheduling software. It was a symphony of precision, each appointment slotted with the care of a skilled composer. In the heart of the bustling ambulatory care clinic, this delicate dance of scheduling was the lifeblood that kept the facility running smoothly, ensuring that every patient received the attention they deserved.

As the day unfolded, the receptionist's desk became a hub of activity, a well-choreographed ballet of phone calls, form-filling, and computer keystrokes. With a warm smile and a soothing tone, she listened to the needs of each patient, carefully assessing their situation and guiding them towards the most suitable appointment times. She understood that every person who walked through the doors was unique, with their own story, their own concerns, and their own challenges – and it was her job to weave those individual threads into a harmonious tapestry of care.

The key to this efficiency lay in the clinic's meticulously crafted scheduling system, a digital symphony that seamlessly coordinated the availability of providers, the needs of patients, and the flow of the clinic itself. By leveraging the power of technology, the receptionist could swiftly identify open slots, prioritize urgent cases, and ensure that the clinic's resources were utilized to their fullest. Gone were the days of handwritten schedules and endless phone tag – this was a world where the click of a mouse and the stroke of a keyboard could unlock the secrets of efficient patient management.

But it was not merely the technology that made this system a success. The clinic had invested time and effort into crafting a comprehensive scheduling strategy, one that took into account the unique needs of their patient population, the availability of their providers, and the ebb and flow of demand. By analyzing historical data, they were able to identify patterns and anticipate the busiest times, allowing them to allocate resources accordingly and minimize the risk of overbooking or long wait times.

At the heart of this strategy was a deep understanding of patient priorities. The receptionist knew that for some, the convenience of an early morning or late afternoon appointment was paramount, while for others, the need for prompt attention to an acute concern took precedence. By carefully listening to each patient's needs and preferences, she was able to find the perfect balance, ensuring that everyone left the clinic feeling satisfied and cared for.

But the true magic of this scheduling system lay in its ability to adapt and evolve. As the clinic's patient population grew and the demands on its services changed, the scheduling team remained vigilant, constantly refining their processes and exploring new technologies to keep up with the ever-shifting landscape of healthcare. It was a delicate dance, a constant ebb and flow of adjustments and fine-tuning, but one that ultimately paid dividends in the form of satisfied patients and a well-oiled clinical operation.

And so, as the day drew to a close and the last patient bid farewell, the receptionist allowed herself a moment of quiet reflection. She knew that her role was more than just a series of keystrokes and phone calls – it was the orchestration of a complex and vital system, one that ensured that every person who walked through the clinic's doors received the care and attention they deserved. It was a responsibility she took to heart, a calling that filled her with a sense of purpose and pride. For in the end, the true measure of a successful scheduling system was not just the efficiency of its operations, but the impact it had on the lives of those it served – and that was a legacy she was proud to be a part of.

Environmental Safety Issues in Ambulatory Care

As the sun peeked through the window, casting a warm glow across the bustling ambulatory care clinic, the nurses gathered for their morning briefing. With gentle smiles and a touch of whimsy, they discussed the day's environmental safety considerations, armed with a keen sense of purpose and a commitment to creating a haven of comfort and security for their patients.

Infection control was at the forefront of their minds, for they knew that the delicate balance of a healing environment hinged on their vigilance. With a touch of practiced efficiency, the nurses reviewed the protocols for hand hygiene, surface disinfection, and the proper usage of personal protective equipment. Their words flowed like a soothing melody, reassuring patients and colleagues alike that their wellbeing was of the utmost importance.

As the day unfolded, the nurses deftly navigated the intricate dance of emergency preparedness. They spoke in hushed tones, sharing strategies for responding to a wide range of potential scenarios, from natural disasters to medical emergencies. Their voices carried a hint of calm determination, instilling a sense of confidence and trust in all who occupied the clinic's halls.

With each patient interaction, the nurses wove a tapestry of tranquility and comfort. They moved with a graceful rhythm, mindful of the sensory needs of their patients, carefully adjusting lighting, temperature, and ambient noise to create a serene environment. The soft touch of their hands, the gentle lilt of their voices, and the genuine warmth of their smiles all combined to soothe the anxious hearts of those who sought their care.

In the quiet moments between appointments, the nurses reflected on the importance of their roles as stewards of environmental safety. They knew that the success of their clinic's mission hinged on their ability to anticipate and address the unique needs of each patient, from the frail elderly to the curious children. With a collective sense of pride and purpose, they committed themselves to continuously improving their practices, staying attuned to the latest research and best practices in ambulatory care nursing.

As the day drew to a close, the nurses gathered once more, their voices mingling in a soft chorus of shared experiences and insights. They spoke of the challenges they had navigated, the triumphs they had celebrated, and the endless opportunities to enhance the safety and wellbeing of their patients. With a touch of whimsy and a deep well of compassion, they knew that their work was not just a profession, but a calling – a chance to create a sanctuary of healing and comfort, one patient at a time.

Conflict Resolution in Ambulatory Care

The waiting room buzzed with a low murmur as patients shuffled quietly, glancing at the clock and fidgeting with magazines. In the hallway, the air carried a touch of tension, a quiet undercurrent of unease that no one dared to acknowledge. But Samantha, the head nurse, knew what lay beneath the surface—the occasional clashes and conflicts that arose in the fast-paced world of ambulatory care.

With a gentle smile, Samantha made her way through the clinic, her steps quiet and assured. She paused at the nurse's station, taking a moment to observe the rhythmic flow of the day. Nurses and medical assistants moved with practiced efficiency, attending to patients, processing paperwork, and coordinating care. But Samantha knew that beneath this veneer of order, the potential for conflict was ever-present.

It was her role, as the seasoned leader, to ensure that any disruptions were addressed swiftly and effectively. Conflict, if left unresolved, had a way of festering, affecting morale, productivity, and most importantly, the quality of patient care. Samantha took a deep breath, preparing to impart her wealth of knowledge on the topic to her team.

Gathering the staff for a brief meeting, Samantha's soothing voice cut through the chatter. "It's important that we all understand the art of conflict resolution," she began, her gaze sweeping the room. "In the fast-paced world of ambulatory care, tensions can arise, and it's our responsibility to navigate these challenges with grace and empathy."

Samantha emphasized the importance of effective communication, stressing the need to listen attentively, speak with clarity, and avoid making assumptions. "When conflicts arise, it's crucial that we approach the situation with an open mind and a willingness to understand the other person's perspective," she said, her voice warm and inviting.

The nurses nodded in agreement, their eyes reflecting the weight of Samantha's words. They knew all too well the consequences of poor communication—misunderstandings that snowballed into full-blown arguments, strained relationships, and ultimately, disruptions in patient care.

Samantha then delved into the art of negotiation, reminding her team that the goal was not to win, but to find a mutually beneficial solution. "Compromise and collaboration are the keys to effective conflict resolution," she said, her hands gesturing gently. "We must be willing to listen, to find common ground, and to work together towards a resolution that satisfies all parties."

The nurses leaned in, their attention rapt, as Samantha shared real-life examples of how she had navigated challenging situations in the past. She spoke of the time a physician had clashed with a medical assistant over a patient's treatment plan, and how she had facilitated a respectful dialogue that ultimately led to a better course of action. She recounted the incident where two nurses had disagreed over the best way to handle a particularly difficult patient, and how she had guided them to find a compromise that worked for everyone.

Throughout her guidance, Samantha emphasized the importance of maintaining a calm and professional demeanor, even in the face of heated emotions. "It's easy to get caught up in the intensity of the moment," she acknowledged, "but it's our responsibility to remain level-headed and focused on finding a solution."

As the meeting drew to a close, Samantha reminded her team that a collaborative and respectful work environment was not only essential for their own well-being, but also for the well-being of their patients. "When we work together, when we communicate effectively and resolve conflicts with empathy and grace, we create a space where everyone can thrive," she said, her gaze warm and encouraging.

The nurses left the meeting with a renewed sense of purpose, their steps lighter and their spirits buoyed by Samantha's words. They knew that in the ever-evolving world of ambulatory care, conflicts would inevitably arise, but they were now better equipped to handle them with the care and professionalism that their patients deserved.

Delegation of Duties in Ambulatory Care

In the warm embrace of the ambulatory care clinic, the gentle hum of efficiency and the soothing flow of patient care create an atmosphere of calm and purpose. It is within this delicate balance that the delegation of duties becomes a dance, a graceful interplay of skills, responsibilities, and the unwavering commitment to ensure each patient's well-being.

As the sun's rays filter through the windows, casting a soft glow upon the bustling clinic, the nurse leader, a beacon of experience and wisdom, takes a moment to pause and reflect. With a serene smile, they recognize the importance of thoughtful delegation, a cornerstone of successful ambulatory care nursing. For it is through the harmonious delegation of tasks that the team can truly shine, each member contributing their unique talents to the greater good of the patients they serve.

Legal and Ethical Considerations

In the realm of ambulatory care, where every interaction carries the weight of trust and responsibility, the delegation of duties is not merely a logistical exercise, but a delicate dance guided by the principles of law and ethics. The nurse leader, like a conductor orchestrating a symphony, must navigate the intricate web of regulations and professional standards, ensuring that each member of the team operates within their scope of practice and maintains the highest levels of patient safety and quality of care.

With a keen eye for detail and a deep understanding of the legal landscape, the nurse leader carefully crafts a delegation plan that not only maximizes efficiency but also safeguards the rights and well-being of both patients and staff. Every decision is made with the utmost consideration, balancing the unique needs of the clinic, the expertise of the team, and the unwavering commitment to upholding the ethical principles that govern the nursing profession.

Delegation Principles

As the nurse leader weaves the intricate tapestry of delegation, they draw upon a set of time-honored principles that serve as the foundation for their approach. Like a gardener tending to a flourishing garden, they understand that the key to successful delegation lies in the intentional selection and nurturing of the right tasks for the right team members.

With a discerning eye, the nurse leader assesses the skills, knowledge, and capabilities of each member of the team, matching their strengths and areas of expertise to the specific tasks at hand. This thoughtful pairing not only ensures optimal patient care but also fosters a sense of empowerment and growth within the team, as each individual is given the opportunity to contribute in meaningful and fulfilling ways.

Equally important is the clear communication of expectations and the provision of adequate resources and support. The nurse leader, like a gentle mentor, guides the team, ensuring that everyone understands their roles, responsibilities, and the desired outcomes. This collaborative approach instills a sense of confidence and ownership, empowering each team member to take on their delegated tasks with a renewed sense of purpose and determination.

Strategies for Effective Delegation

In the ever-evolving landscape of ambulatory care, the nurse leader must be a creative problem-solver, constantly adapting their delegation strategies to meet the changing needs of the clinic and its patients. With a touch of whimsy and a keen eye for detail, they weave together a tapestry of effective delegation that is both practical and inspirational.

One such strategy is the implementation of cross-training, where team members are encouraged to develop a versatile skillset, able to adapt to the ebb and flow of the clinic's demands. This not only fosters a sense of interdependence and collaboration but also allows the nurse leader to seamlessly redistribute tasks as needed, ensuring that the patient's journey remains uninterrupted and the team's productivity remains high.

Another key approach is the establishment of clear communication channels, where team members feel empowered to voice their concerns, ask questions, and provide feedback. The nurse leader, like a gentle guiding light, creates an environment of trust and open dialogue, where everyone's contributions are valued and respected. This collaborative spirit not only enhances the effectiveness of delegation but also cultivates a sense of camaraderie and shared purpose within the team.

Finally, the nurse leader embraces the power of technology, leveraging digital tools and platforms to streamline the delegation process and enhance the team's efficiency. From automated task management systems to real-time communication platforms, these innovative solutions help to minimize the burden of administrative tasks, allowing the team to focus on the essence of their work - delivering exceptional patient care.

In the end, the delegation of duties in ambulatory care nursing is not merely a practical necessity, but a testament to the nurse leader's unwavering commitment to the well-being of both patients and staff. Through a delicate balance of legal and ethical considerations, carefully curated delegation principles, and a repertoire of innovative strategies, the nurse leader weaves a tapestry of success, where every team member shines brightly, and the patient's journey is marked by the finest quality of care.

Managed Care Plans in Ambulatory Care

As the sun gently dipped below the horizon, casting a warm glow over the bustling ambulatory care clinic, the nurses gathered for their weekly meeting. The air was filled with a palpable sense of purpose, as they discussed the ever-evolving landscape of managed care plans and their role in ensuring seamless, high-quality patient care.

The head nurse, Sarah, began the meeting with a gentle smile, her voice soothing and inviting. "Our patients are at the heart of everything we do, and it's our responsibility to navigate the complexities of managed care plans with the utmost care and attention," she said, her words carrying a quiet authority.

As the nurses listened intently, Sarah outlined the different types of managed care models that they encountered in their daily practice. "From health maintenance organizations (HMOs) to preferred provider organizations (PPOs) and point-of-service (POS) plans, each model has its own unique set of guidelines and reimbursement structures," she explained, her hands gesturing gracefully to illustrate her points.

The nurses nodded in understanding, their eyes shining with a renewed sense of purpose. They knew that navigating these intricate systems was crucial in ensuring their patients received the care they needed, without unnecessary financial burden.

Sarah continued, her voice soothing and reassuring. "As ambulatory care nurses, we play a vital role in coordinating care within the managed care framework. From guiding patients through the maze of provider networks to advocating for the most appropriate treatments and services, our attention to detail and commitment to patient advocacy are paramount."

The nurses murmured in agreement, inspired by Sarah's words and the shared conviction that their work made a genuine difference in the lives of their patients.

Transitioning to the topic of reimbursement systems, Sarah explained the complexities of negotiating with managed care organizations to ensure fair and timely compensation for the services they provided. "It's a delicate balance, ensuring that our patients receive the care they need while also securing the necessary funding to sustain our practice," she said, her brow furrowing slightly with the weight of the responsibility.

The nurses listened intently, their fingers tapping thoughtfully on the tabletops as they considered the nuances of this challenge. They knew that their role extended beyond the clinical realm, and that navigating the financial aspects of managed care was an integral part of their responsibilities.

As the meeting drew to a close, Sarah's gaze swept across the room, her eyes filled with a quiet pride. "Remember, my dear colleagues, that our work is a symphony of compassion, skill, and dedication. Let us continue to be the guiding lights that illuminate the path for our patients, ever-vigilant in our pursuit of holistic, high-quality care."

The nurses nodded in agreement, their spirits lifted by Sarah's words. With renewed energy and a steadfast commitment to their patients, they exited the room, ready to face the challenges and opportunities that the world of managed care would bring.

Performance Improvement in Ambulatory Care

The soft patter of footsteps echoed through the sunlit halls of the ambulatory care center, a gentle rhythm punctuated by the occasional murmur of voices and the gentle hum of medical equipment. Here, in this oasis of care, a dedicated team of nurses tended to the needs of their patients with unwavering focus and a touch of quiet magic.

At the heart of this harmonious dance lay the pursuit of performance improvement – a delicate balance of data analysis, quality assessment, and the seamless integration of evidence-based practices. It was a journey of continuous refinement, where every step was guided by a deep understanding of the needs of both patients and healthcare providers.

Frances, the lead nurse of the ambulatory care unit, often likened the process to that of a master gardener, carefully tending to the intricate web of factors that contributed to the flourishing of her patients' well-being. With a keen eye and a gentle hand, she and her team meticulously examined the data, seeking out the subtle patterns and insights that would guide their efforts.

In the serene confines of the nurses' station, Frances would gather her colleagues, their faces aglow with the warm light filtering through the windows. Together, they would pore over the reports, discussing the trends and identifying areas where improvements could be made. It was a dance of collaboration, each nurse offering their unique perspective, their collective wisdom shaping the path forward.

Time and again, Frances marveled at the power of data – how the seemingly mundane numbers and statistics could unlock the secrets to enhanced patient outcomes and streamlined healthcare delivery. With a touch of wonder, she watched as her team transformed these insights into tangible actions, implementing evidence-based practices that brought a sense of calm and comfort to the lives of their patients.

In the cozy examination rooms, the nurses moved with a practiced grace, their movements choreographed to perfection. They listened intently to the concerns of their patients, offering a gentle, reassuring presence that put even the most anxious souls at ease. And as they implemented the carefully crafted protocols, the nurses' touch carried with it a hint of whimsy, a soothing balm that soothed both body and spirit.

The true magic, however, unfolded in the subtle moments – the lingering smile exchanged with a nervous patient, the soft-spoken words of encouragement that lifted a heavy heart, the tender touch that conveyed a depth of understanding beyond mere words. It was in these fleeting, yet profound, interactions that the true essence of performance improvement was revealed – a tapestry of compassion, expertise, and an unwavering commitment to the well-being of those entrusted to their care.

As the sun dipped low on the horizon, casting a warm glow over the bustling center, Frances would pause for a moment, her gaze sweeping over the scene with a profound sense of pride and fulfillment. In this haven of healing, her team had woven a delicate tapestry of excellence, each thread a testament to their dedication and the transformative power of performance improvement. And as she turned to face the dawn of a new day, Frances knew that the journey had only just begun, filled with endless possibilities for growth, innovation, and the continued betterment of the lives they touched.

5

ADVANCING EDUCATION IN AMBULATORY CARE

Health Promotion and Health Education

In the softly-lit clinic, the soothing melody of the wind chimes drifted through the air, carrying a gentle reminder of the importance of holistic well-being. Nurse Emily, her warm smile reflecting the tranquility of the space, welcomed each patient with a compassionate approach, her every interaction a gentle invitation to embark on a journey toward healthier living.

As the patients settled into the cozy armchairs, Nurse Emily began her rounds, her steps light and her gaze attentive. With a nurturing touch, she listened to their concerns, her soothing voice guiding them through the maze of health information, empowering them to take an active role in their own care.

"Today, we'll explore the art of living well," she said, her words flowing like a gentle stream. "Together, we'll discover the small, yet profound, steps we can take to nourish our bodies, minds, and spirits – for it is in this delicate balance that true health blossoms."

Nurse Emily's patients leaned in, captivated by her gentle wisdom. With a touch of whimsy, she wove together the tapestry of healthy living, highlighting the importance of nutrition, physical activity, and stress management. She spoke of the wonder of the human body, guiding her patients to a deeper understanding of their own unique needs and capabilities.

As she moved through the clinic, Nurse Emily carried with her a sense of lightness and joy, her presence a soothing balm for the weary souls who sought her care. She encouraged her patients to explore the natural world, to find solace in the simple pleasures of a brisk walk or a mindful moment in the garden.

"Our bodies are remarkable, resilient beings," she said, her eyes sparkling with wonder. "When we nourish them with wholesome foods, gentle movements, and moments of calm, we unlock the door to a life filled with vitality and joy."

Carefully, Nurse Emily introduced her patients to a wealth of educational resources – from informative pamphlets to interactive workshops – each one designed to empower them to take an active role in their health. She encouraged them to ask questions, to seek out the information that resonated most deeply with their individual needs and preferences.

"There is no one-size-fits-all approach to wellness," she explained, her voice soft and reassuring. "Each of us is unique, with our own gifts and challenges. The key is to approach our health with compassion, to listen to the wisdom of our bodies, and to celebrate the small steps we take each day."

As the patients left the clinic, their steps a little lighter, their minds a little clearer, they carried with them the seeds of transformation. Nurse Emily's gentle guidance had inspired them to consider new possibilities, to dream of a future where their well-being was not just a distant goal, but a vibrant, tangible reality.

In the days that followed, the patients would return, eager to share their progress and eager to learn more. And Nurse Emily, with her infinite patience and her boundless empathy, would be there to greet them, ready to walk alongside them on their journey toward a healthier, more fulfilling life.

Applying Social Cognitive Theory in Ambulatory Care

Nestled within the quiet halls of the ambulatory care clinic, a gentle rhythm unfolds. Patients trickle in, their faces reflecting a blend of apprehension and hope. It is here, in this serene sanctuary, that the principles of Social Cognitive Theory come to life, guiding nurses in their quest to empower individuals on their journey towards better health.

As the sun filters through the windows, casting a warm glow, the nurses greet each patient with a soft smile and a genuine interest in their well-being. They understand that true transformation begins not with lectures or directives, but with a profound connection that fosters trust and understanding.

At the heart of their approach lies the concept of self-efficacy – the belief that one has the ability to achieve desired outcomes. Nurses versed in Social Cognitive Theory recognize that this belief is the foundation upon which lasting change is built. Through the art of motivational interviewing, they gently guide patients in exploring their own strengths, uncovering their intrinsic motivations, and envisioning a future where healthier choices become the natural course of action.

With a deft touch, the nurses weave a tapestry of encouragement and empowerment. They listen intently, capturing the nuances of each patient's story, and then reflect back their observations with a keen understanding. This collaborative process enables patients to see themselves not as passive recipients of care, but as active participants in their own transformation.

As the session unfolds, the nurses deftly navigate the complexities of behavior change models, tailoring their approach to the unique needs and readiness of each individual. They understand that change is not a linear path, but a journey with ebbs and flows, and they are ready to provide the necessary support and guidance along the way.

With a gentle touch and a calming presence, the nurses guide their patients through the exploration of barriers and the identification of achievable goals. They help them visualize success, cultivating a sense of self-confidence that ripples outward, empowering patients to take the first steps towards a healthier future.

In the quiet moments between appointments, the nurses reflect on the small but significant victories they have witnessed. A patient who has finally mustered the courage to quit smoking, another who has discovered the joy of incorporating more physical activity into their daily routine – these are the moments that fuel their passion and reinforce the power of Social Cognitive Theory in action.

As the day draws to a close, the nurses take a moment to savor the sense of accomplishment that comes with their work. They know that the transformation they have witnessed is not just a change in behavior, but a shift in mindset – a newfound belief in the individual's capacity to shape their own destiny.

In the ambulatory care setting, the application of Social Cognitive Theory has become a beacon of hope, illuminating the path towards lasting, meaningful change. Through the gentle guidance and unwavering support of these compassionate nurses, patients are empowered to take charge of their health, one small step at a time, and to embrace a future filled with possibilities.

Community Health Initiatives in Ambulatory Care

The sun gently filters through the windows, casting a warm glow upon the bustling community center. Soft laughter and the gentle hum of conversation fill the air, as a group of eager residents gather to learn about the latest health initiative. In the corner, a nurse stands ready, her kind eyes and welcoming smile instantly putting everyone at ease.

This is the heart of ambulatory care nursing - a world where the boundaries between the clinic and the community blur, and the nurse becomes a beacon of hope, guiding individuals towards healthier, more fulfilling lives. It is a realm where the nurse's role extends far beyond the confines of the examination room, encompassing the promotion of wellness, the forging of partnerships, and the championing of diverse healthcare needs.

At the center of this vibrant tapestry are the health promotion programs that the ambulatory care nurse so diligently weaves. These programs, like delicate threads, are carefully tailored to the unique needs and cultural preferences of the community, creating a tapestry of well-being that is both inclusive and empowering.

Take, for instance, the recently launched diabetes education workshop. Recognizing the high prevalence of the condition within the local Hispanic population, the nurse collaborated with community leaders to design a program that not only imparts essential knowledge but also celebrates the rich culinary traditions of the community. Participants gather, not just to learn about meal planning and medication management, but to share cherished family recipes, swap stories, and discover the joy of healthy, culturally-relevant cooking.

In another corner of the community center, a group of young mothers gathers for a prenatal yoga class, led by a compassionate nurse who understands the unique challenges faced by expectant women. The gentle movements and soothing breaths are accompanied by soft music and encouraging words, creating a nurturing environment where the women can find solace, support, and the confidence to navigate the journey of motherhood.

But the reach of the ambulatory care nurse extends far beyond the confines of the community center. Through strategic partnerships with local organizations, schools, and faith-based institutions, these healthcare advocates forge connections that amplify the impact of their work. By aligning with trusted community leaders and leveraging shared resources, they are able to identify and address the pressing healthcare needs of diverse populations, from the elderly seeking assistance with chronic disease management to the marginalized youth in need of mental health support.

One such partnership, forged between the ambulatory care clinic and a nearby senior living facility, has resulted in a thriving "Healthy Aging" program. Every week, the nurse visits the facility, offering check-ups, educational workshops, and one-on-one consultations to the residents. The program has not only improved the physical well-being of the participants but has also fostered a sense of community, as the seniors share their stories, support one another, and find renewed purpose in their golden years.

In these moments, the ambulatory care nurse transcends the role of a mere healthcare provider, becoming a trusted confidante, a compassionate listener, and a champion of holistic well-being. Whether guiding a young mother through the joys and challenges of pregnancy, or empowering a senior to manage their chronic condition with confidence, the nurse's impact ripples outward, touching the lives of individuals and the community as a whole.

As the sun sets, casting a warm glow over the community center, the nurse pauses to reflect on the day's work. The faces of those she has helped, the stories she has heard, and the connections she has forged all serve as a gentle reminder of the profound impact that ambulatory care nursing can have. With a renewed sense of purpose, she turns her gaze towards the horizon, eager to continue weaving the tapestry of community health, one thread at a time.

Embracing Cultural Diversity in Ambulatory Care

As the sun peeked through the window, casting a warm glow across the cozy waiting room, Nurse Emma greeted her first patient of the day with a gentle smile. Amelia, a young woman from a diverse cultural background, approached the check-in desk, her eyes conveying a sense of apprehension. Emma, ever-mindful of the importance of cultural sensitivity, welcomed Amelia with open arms, guiding her through the check-in process with a soothing tone and a keen understanding of her unique needs.

At the heart of ambulatory care nursing lies the unwavering commitment to providing personalized, culturally-responsive care to individuals from all walks of life. In this ever-evolving landscape of healthcare, where diversity is the thread that binds communities together, it is essential for nurses to cultivate a deep appreciation for the richness and complexity of cultural differences.

As Amelia settled into the examination room, Emma began her assessment, taking the time to listen attentively and ask thoughtful questions. She recognized that Amelia's cultural background might shape her perceptions of health, illness, and the healthcare system itself. By approaching the interaction with empathy and a genuine desire to understand, Emma ensured that Amelia felt heard, respected, and at ease.

Cultural competence, the foundation of effective ambulatory care, is not merely a set of skills to be acquired; it is a lifelong journey of self-reflection, learning, and active engagement with diverse communities. Nurses must be willing to step outside their own cultural frames of reference, recognize their own biases, and continuously expand their knowledge and understanding of the beliefs, traditions, and practices that shape the lives of their patients.

Through this process of cultural exploration, nurses can become adept at navigating the complexities of healthcare interactions, recognizing and addressing health disparities, and tailoring their approach to the unique needs of each patient. By embracing the richness of cultural diversity, they can foster an environment of trust, open communication, and collaborative decision-making – the cornerstones of holistic, patient-centered care.

As Amelia's appointment progressed, Emma deftly wove her cultural awareness into the care plan, suggesting gentle modifications to accommodate Amelia's preferences and beliefs. She explained medical concepts in a manner that resonated with Amelia's cultural understanding, ensuring that the information was accessible and meaningful. This attentiveness to cultural nuances not only put Amelia at ease but also empowered her to take an active role in her own healthcare journey.

In the world of ambulatory care, where patients often navigate the healthcare system independently, the need for culturally sensitive nursing practices becomes even more paramount. Nurses must be equipped to address the unique challenges faced by individuals from diverse backgrounds, such as language barriers, health literacy gaps, and disparities in access to care. By proactively addressing these barriers, nurses can help bridge the divide and ensure that all patients receive the high-quality, equitable care they deserve.

As Amelia's appointment drew to a close, Emma took a moment to reflect on the importance of this encounter. Each patient who walks through the doors of the ambulatory care clinic brings with them a unique cultural tapestry, woven with traditions, beliefs, and lived experiences. By embracing this diversity and fostering an environment of cultural understanding, nurses can not only provide exceptional care but also contribute to the overall well-being of the communities they serve.

In the ever-evolving landscape of healthcare, the role of the ambulatory care nurse as a cultural ambassador and advocate becomes increasingly vital. By continually expanding their knowledge, honing their communication skills, and cultivating a deep respect for cultural differences, these nurses can truly make a lasting impact on the lives of their patients, one heartfelt interaction at a time.

Primary, Secondary, and Tertiary Health Prevention

In the gentle embrace of the ambulatory care setting, the nurse's role shines as a beacon of preventive care. Here, where the rhythms of everyday life meet the pursuit of wellness, a tapestry of health promotion unfolds, woven with the threads of primary, secondary, and tertiary prevention.

Picture a serene morning in the clinic, the air filled with the soft murmurs of patients and the reassuring presence of the nursing staff. It is here, amidst the quiet hum of activity, that the nurse's keen eye and compassionate heart begin their work, guiding individuals towards a future of vibrant health.

Primary prevention, like a delicate seedling, takes root in this nurturing environment. The nurse, a gentle gardener, sows the seeds of education and awareness, empowering patients to cultivate their own well-being. With a touch of whimsy and a steady hand, they share the wisdom of healthy lifestyles, from the importance of regular exercise to the joys of nutritious meals. Through these conversations, the nurse becomes a trusted companion, walking alongside patients as they embark on their journeys towards wellness.

As the sun rises higher in the sky, the nurse's focus shifts to the realm of secondary prevention – a realm where early detection and timely intervention can make all the difference. With a keen eye and a compassionate spirit, the nurse guides patients through the myriad of health screenings, each one a gentle exploration of the body's secrets. Whether it's a routine mammogram or a blood pressure check, the nurse's deft touch and soothing presence transform these moments into opportunities for connection and reassurance.

In this dance of prevention, the nurse becomes a master storyteller, weaving together the threads of the patient's health history and the subtle signals of the body. With each screening, a new chapter unfolds, revealing the potential for early intervention and the promise of a brighter future. It is in these moments that the nurse's role truly shines, as they gently guide patients towards the path of proactive care, empowering them to take an active role in their own well-being.

Yet, the nurse's tapestry of preventive care does not end there. Tertiary prevention, the final strands, requires a delicate touch and a deep well of compassion. Here, the nurse becomes a guiding light for those facing chronic conditions or the aftermath of acute illness, offering support, education, and a gentle hand to navigate the complexities of ongoing management.

With a soothing tone and a keen understanding, the nurse helps patients reframe their challenges, transforming them into opportunities for growth and resilience. They share the secrets of self-care, unveiling the power of mindfulness, gentle exercise, and the healing embrace of a supportive community. In these moments, the nurse becomes a beacon of hope, illuminating the path towards a life of renewed vitality and quality.

As the day draws to a close and the clinic settles into the tranquil hush of the evening, the nurse's work continues, a tapestry of preventive care woven with threads of empathy, education, and the unwavering commitment to the well-being of those entrusted to their care. It is a symphony of small moments, each one a testament to the nurse's ability to transform lives, one gentle step at a time.

Research Methodologies in Ambulatory Care

As the sun rises gently over the bustling city, the quiet halls of the ambulatory care clinic come alive with the soft patter of footsteps and the gentle hum of conversation. This is where the true magic of healthcare happens – where patients are nurtured back to health with a personal touch, and where nurses, armed with the latest research and evidence-based practices, work tirelessly to improve the well-being of their community.

In the serene confines of the clinic, the research methodologies employed by the dedicated nursing staff play a crucial role in shaping the future of patient care. From the delicate design of observational studies to the robust analysis of patient data, each step in the research process is imbued with a sense of purpose and a commitment to excellence.

As the morning light filters through the windows, the nurses gather, their minds abuzz with the possibilities that lie ahead. They know that the path to better patient outcomes is paved with rigorous investigation and a deep understanding of the unique challenges faced by those they serve. With a touch of whimsy and a generous dose of compassion, they embark on their research journey, guided by the principles of evidence-based practice.

The first step in this odyssey is the careful selection of study designs. Whether they choose to delve into the intricacies of randomized controlled trials or the nuances of qualitative case studies, the nurses understand that the foundation of their research must be solid and well-crafted. They meticulously plan their data collection methods, ensuring that every touchpoint with their patients is infused with a sense of care and empathy.

As the day unfolds, the nurses immerse themselves in the rich tapestry of patient experiences, gathering insights that will shape the future of their practice. They listen intently, their senses alive to the subtle cues that whisper of the unique needs and preferences of each individual. With a gentle touch and a soothing tone, they coax forth the stories that will inform their research, weaving together a tapestry of lived experiences that will serve as the bedrock of their findings.

In the quiet moments between patient visits, the nurses retreat to their research stations, their fingers dancing across the keyboards as they meticulously analyze the data they have collected. They pour over the numbers, searching for patterns and trends that will illuminate the path forward. With a keen eye for detail and a deep understanding of statistical methods, they uncover insights that will inform their practice and transform the lives of their patients.

As the sun sets and the clinic falls silent, the nurses reflect on the day's work, their hearts filled with a sense of purpose and a deep commitment to the principles of evidence-based practice. They know that their research is not just a means to an end, but a living, breathing extension of their dedication to the well-being of their community. With a touch of whimsy and a spark of innovation, they look forward to the next day, eager to continue their journey of discovery and to bring the power of research to the forefront of ambulatory care.

The Role of Clinical Pathways in Ambulatory Care

In the ever-evolving landscape of healthcare, the role of clinical pathways has become increasingly crucial in the realm of ambulatory care nursing. These standardized care plans not only streamline the delivery of care but also foster interdisciplinary collaboration, ultimately improving patient outcomes and care coordination.

The development and implementation of clinical pathways in ambulatory care settings serve as a strategic framework for nurses to navigate the complexities of patient management. By outlining evidence-based best practices, these pathways provide a structured approach to care, ensuring that patients receive consistent and high-quality services across different healthcare settings.

One of the key advantages of clinical pathways in ambulatory care is their ability to promote interdisciplinary collaboration. Nurses, physicians, therapists, and other healthcare professionals work together to align their efforts, sharing their expertise and insights to create a comprehensive care plan tailored to the unique needs of each patient. This collaborative approach enhances communication, reduces fragmentation, and ensures that all team members are working towards the same patient-centered goals.

The integration of clinical pathways in ambulatory care has also demonstrated its efficacy in improving care coordination. By standardizing the care process, nurses can seamlessly transition patients between different levels of care, streamlining the continuum of care and minimizing the risk of gaps or delays. This seamless coordination not only enhances the patient experience but also reduces the likelihood of adverse events and readmissions, ultimately leading to better patient outcomes.

Moreover, the implementation of clinical pathways in ambulatory care settings has been shown to have a positive impact on resource utilization and cost-effectiveness. By guiding healthcare professionals in the most efficient use of resources, such as diagnostic tests, interventions, and follow-up appointments, clinical pathways can help optimize the allocation of limited healthcare resources and reduce unnecessary expenditures.

Developing and implementing effective clinical pathways in ambulatory care requires a multifaceted approach. Nurses play a crucial role in this process, collaborating with interdisciplinary teams to identify evidence-based best practices, define key performance indicators, and continuously monitor and refine the pathways to ensure their effectiveness.

The success of clinical pathways in ambulatory care hinges on the ability of nurses to effectively communicate the benefits of these standardized care plans to patients and their families. By educating patients on the purpose and expected outcomes of the clinical pathway, nurses can foster a shared understanding and promote greater patient engagement, ultimately leading to improved adherence and better health outcomes.

In conclusion, the role of clinical pathways in ambulatory care nursing is undeniable. By promoting interdisciplinary collaboration, enhancing care coordination, and optimizing resource utilization, these standardized care plans have the potential to transform the delivery of healthcare, ensuring that patients receive the highest quality of care in the most efficient and cost-effective manner.

In the ever-evolving landscape of healthcare, the role of clinical pathways has become increasingly crucial in the realm of ambulatory care nursing. These standardized care plans not only streamline the delivery of care but also foster interdisciplinary collaboration, ultimately improving patient outcomes and care coordination.

The development and implementation of clinical pathways in ambulatory care settings serve as a strategic framework for nurses to navigate the complexities of patient management. By outlining evidence-based best practices, these pathways provide a structured approach to care, ensuring that patients receive consistent and high-quality services across different healthcare settings.

One of the key advantages of clinical pathways in ambulatory care is their ability to promote interdisciplinary collaboration. Nurses, physicians, therapists, and other healthcare professionals work together to align their efforts, sharing their expertise and insights to create a comprehensive care plan tailored to the unique needs of each patient. This collaborative approach enhances communication, reduces fragmentation, and ensures that all team members are working towards the same patient-centered goals.

The integration of clinical pathways in ambulatory care has also demonstrated its efficacy in improving care coordination. By standardizing the care process, nurses can seamlessly transition patients between different levels of care, streamlining the continuum of care and minimizing the risk of gaps or delays. This seamless coordination not only enhances the patient experience but also reduces the likelihood of adverse events and readmissions, ultimately leading to better patient outcomes.

Moreover, the implementation of clinical pathways in ambulatory care settings has been shown to have a positive impact on resource utilization and cost-effectiveness. By guiding healthcare professionals in the most efficient use of resources, such as diagnostic tests, interventions, and follow-up appointments, clinical pathways can help optimize the allocation of limited healthcare resources and reduce unnecessary expenditures.

Developing and implementing effective clinical pathways in ambulatory care requires a multifaceted approach. Nurses play a crucial role in this process, collaborating with interdisciplinary teams to identify evidence-based best practices, define key performance indicators, and continuously monitor and refine the pathways to ensure their effectiveness.

The success of clinical pathways in ambulatory care hinges on the ability of nurses to effectively communicate the benefits of these standardized care plans to patients and their families. By educating patients on the purpose and expected outcomes of the clinical pathway, nurses can foster a shared understanding and promote greater patient engagement, ultimately leading to improved adherence and better health outcomes.

In conclusion, the role of clinical pathways in ambulatory care nursing is undeniable. By promoting interdisciplinary collaboration, enhancing care coordination, and optimizing resource utilization, these standardized care plans have the potential to transform the delivery of healthcare, ensuring that patients receive the highest quality of care in the most efficient and cost-effective manner.

In the gentle embrace of the ambulatory care setting, where the rhythm of everyday life blends seamlessly with the art of healing, the role of clinical pathways emerges as a guiding light. These meticulously crafted roadmaps, woven with the threads of interdisciplinary collaboration, hold the promise of elevating the patient experience and fostering exceptional care coordination.

As the sun's soft glow filters through the windows, the ambulatory care nursing team gathers, their faces alight with a sense of purpose. The development of these clinical pathways, like the unfurling of a delicate tapestry, requires a harmonious dance of expertise, creativity, and a deep understanding of the unique needs of each patient who walks through the doors.

With a steady hand and an unwavering commitment, the nurses, physicians, and allied health professionals work in tandem, their individual contributions melding into a cohesive whole. They meticulously craft these standardized care plans, each step designed to address the patient's unique journey, from the moment they step into the clinic to the moment they return home, their needs addressed with the utmost care and attention.

As the clinical pathways take shape, the team imbues them with a touch of whimsy and charm, weaving in gentle reminders for patients to pause, breathe, and find solace in the small moments of their day. Soft, sensory imagery is woven throughout, inviting patients to engage their senses and find comfort in the soothing language that guides them along the path to wellness.

The implementation of these clinical pathways is a delicate dance, requiring a deep understanding of the nuances of the ambulatory care setting. The nurses, ever vigilant, meticulously monitor the progress of each patient, adapting the care plan as necessary to ensure the best possible outcomes. They work in tandem with the interdisciplinary team, sharing insights, collaborating on challenges, and constantly refining the process to ensure the seamless delivery of care.

As the patients navigate the twists and turns of their healthcare journey, they are enveloped in the embrace of the clinical pathways, feeling a sense of security and comfort in the carefully crafted steps that guide them. The nurses, with their gentle touch and soothing words, become the beacons of reassurance, walking alongside their patients, offering support and encouragement every step of the way.

In the ambulatory care setting, the role of clinical pathways extends far beyond mere efficiency and standardization. These pathways become the threads that weave together the tapestry of compassionate, patient-centered care, where the individual needs of each person are addressed with the utmost care and attention. As the sun sets on another day, the ambulatory care team, with a sense of pride and purpose, reflects on the impact they have made, knowing that their dedication has transformed the lives of those they serve.

6.1 Full-Length Practice Test 1

Section 1: The Clinical Practice

Topic: Focal Points

1. What is a key focal point for ambulatory care nurses when managing chronic diseases?

A) Acute intervention

B) Preventative care

C) Emergency response

D) Medication compliance

Topic: Patient Advocate

2. What role does an ambulatory care nurse play as a patient advocate?

A) Scheduling diagnostic tests

B) Ensuring patient autonomy and informed decision-making

C) Managing the nursing team

D) Approving treatment plans

Topic: Proper Triage

3. Which principle is essential in effective triage within ambulatory care?

A) Treating patients on a first-come, first-served basis

B) Identifying the urgency of a patient's condition

C) Prioritizing based on insurance coverage

D) Referring all cases to specialists

Topic: Qualifications

4. What is a critical qualification required for ambulatory care nurses?

A) Knowledge of inpatient care only

B) Specialization in emergency medicine

C) Proficiency in chronic disease management and patient education

D) Surgical skills

Topic: Care Management

5. In ambulatory care, what is an essential component of care management?

A) Coordinating team schedules

B) Delegating patient responsibilities

C) Integrating multidisciplinary care plans

D) Avoiding patient follow-ups

Section 2: The Communication

Topic: Telehealth Nursing Skills

6. Which skill is crucial for a nurse conducting a telehealth assessment?

A) Physical examination skills

B) Proficient use of verbal and visual cues

C) In-person communication techniques

D) Avoiding patient follow-up

Topic: Documentation

7. What is the primary goal of accurate documentation in ambulatory care?

A) To minimize paperwork

B) To avoid legal repercussions

C) To provide a clear, comprehensive patient care record

D) To reduce the workload of team members

Topic: Cultural Competence

8. What is the first step in providing culturally competent care?

A) Learning a new language

B) Avoiding interaction with diverse patients

C) Recognizing one's own cultural biases

D) Relying only on interpreters

Topic: Service Recovery Process

9. What is an essential step in the service recovery process?

A) Ignoring patient complaints

B) Blaming other team members

C) Acknowledging the patient's concerns and resolving issues promptly

D) Offering financial compensation only

Topic: Informed Consent

10. What must an ambulatory care nurse confirm before obtaining informed consent?

A) The patient has signed the document

B) The patient understands the risks, benefits, and alternatives of the procedure

C) The provider has completed the procedure

D) The family has agreed

Section 3: The Professional Issues

Topic: Licensure Issues

11. What is a primary licensure requirement for ambulatory care nurses?

A) A specialty certificate in emergency medicine

B) An active RN license in good standing

C) A doctoral degree in nursing

D) A temporary nursing license

Topic: Incompetency and Informed Consent

12. When is informed consent invalid?

A) When the patient is under duress

B) When the patient agrees verbally

C) When the provider gives complete details

D) When the patient's guardian consents

Topic: Legal and Ethical Issues

13. What ethical principle is violated when patient confidentiality is breached?

A) Beneficence

B) Non-maleficence

C) Autonomy

D) Justice

Section 3: The Professional Issues

Topic: Skills and Knowledge

14. Which skill is critical for ambulatory care nurses managing complex patient cases?

A) Multitasking without prioritization

B) Advanced critical thinking and decision-making

C) Delegating all care responsibilities

D) Relying only on physician instructions

Topic: Leadership and Management

15. What leadership quality is essential for an ambulatory care nurse manager?

A) Authoritarian decision-making

B) Delegating without supervision

C) Effective communication and team collaboration

D) Avoiding patient interactions

Section 4: The Systems

Topic: Scheduling Patients

16. Which is the best practice for scheduling patients in ambulatory care?

A) Overbooking to accommodate late arrivals

B) Prioritizing based on clinical urgency

C) Scheduling patients with similar conditions together

D) Ignoring follow-up appointments

Topic: Environmental Safety Issues

17. What is a key environmental safety responsibility for an ambulatory care nurse?

A) Performing routine building maintenance

B) Conducting regular safety checks for patient areas

C) Ensuring all medical records are electronic

D) Replacing non-functional equipment only when reported

Topic: Conflict Resolution

18. What is the first step in resolving a conflict between healthcare team members?

A) Ignoring the conflict and continuing work

B) Identifying the root cause of the disagreement

C) Reporting the conflict to senior management immediately

D) Asking the patients for their input

Topic: Delegation of Duties

19. Which task can be appropriately delegated to a licensed practical nurse (LPN)?

A) Patient education about complex procedures

B) Administration of routine medications

C) Independent decision-making for care plans

D) Conducting a detailed initial assessment

Topic: Managed Care Plans

20. What is a primary goal of managed care plans in ambulatory care?

A) Increasing hospital admissions

B) Reducing overall healthcare costs while maintaining quality

C) Limiting patient access to providers

D) Eliminating preventative care services

Section 5: The Education

Topic: Health Promotion and Health Education

21. What is an essential component of health promotion in ambulatory care?

A) Educating patients only during follow-up visits

B) Empowering patients to adopt healthy lifestyle behaviors

C) Avoiding discussions about prevention

D) Focusing solely on medication compliance

Topic: Social Cognitive Theory

22. How can nurses apply Social Cognitive Theory in patient education?

A) By emphasizing punishment for unhealthy behaviors

B) By modeling healthy behaviors and encouraging self-efficacy

C) By disregarding patient beliefs and cultural practices

D) By focusing only on group education

Topic: Community Health

23. What is a primary focus of ambulatory care nurses in community health?

A) Providing inpatient care services

B) Addressing social determinants of health

C) Avoiding involvement in public health initiatives

D) Treating only acute illnesses

Topic: Cultural Diversity

24. How should an ambulatory care nurse approach cultural diversity in patient care?

A) Ignoring cultural differences to ensure uniform care

B) Learning about and respecting each patient's cultural background

C) Assuming all patients have the same healthcare preferences

D) Using a standardized care approach for all

Topic: Primary, Secondary, and Tertiary Health Prevention

25. Which of the following is an example of secondary prevention in ambulatory care?

A) Providing immunizations

B) Conducting regular health screenings

C) Educating patients on smoking cessation

D) Offering rehabilitation services

Section 1: The Clinical Practice

Topic: Focal Points

26. What is a key focus of ambulatory care nurses when addressing patient wellness?

A) Emergency care

B) Prevention and chronic disease management

C) Inpatient treatment

D) Post-surgical rehabilitation

Topic: Patient Advocate

27. How does an ambulatory care nurse act as an advocate during patient education?

A) Dictating the patient's care choices

B) Ensuring the patient fully understands their treatment options

C) Referring patients only to specialists

D) Avoiding discussions about lifestyle changes

Topic: Proper Triage

28. What is the purpose of the triage process in ambulatory care?

A) To ensure all patients are treated simultaneously

B) To determine the order of care based on medical urgency

C) To send all patients to the emergency department

D) To avoid addressing chronic conditions

Topic: Qualifications

29. What additional qualification enhances an ambulatory care nurse's ability to manage complex cases?

A) Certification in telehealth nursing

B) Emergency medical technician (EMT) certification

C) Advanced cardiovascular life support (ACLS) certification

D) Specialization in surgical procedures

Topic: Care Management

30. What is a common tool used in care management for chronic conditions?

A) Patient diaries

B) Randomized scheduling

C) Care management plans tailored to individual needs

D) Emergency-only interventions

Section 2: The Communication

Topic: Telehealth Nursing Skills

31. Which is a critical element of effective communication in telehealth nursing?

A) Ensuring a secure and private communication platform

B) Using only written instructions for patients

C) Avoiding visual aids during video calls

D) Ignoring non-verbal cues

Topic: Documentation

32. Why is real-time documentation considered best practice in ambulatory care?

A) It reduces legal liability completely

B) It allows immediate updates for continuity of care

C) It eliminates the need for follow-up visits

D) It replaces the need for verbal communication

Topic: Cultural Competence

33. What should a nurse do to address language barriers with patients from diverse cultures?

A) Avoid discussing complex topics

B) Use professional medical interpreters

C) Rely solely on family members for translation

D) Assume the patient understands basic terms

Topic: Service Recovery Process

34. What is the final step in an effective service recovery process?

A) Documenting the complaint resolution

B) Apologizing for any issues

C) Ignoring patient concerns

D) Ensuring the problem doesn't happen again

Topic: Informed Consent

35. When is informed consent most effectively obtained?

A) When patients are sedated

B) When the nurse confirms patient comprehension of the procedure

C) After the procedure is completed

D) When only verbal agreement is obtained

Section 3: The Professional Issues

Topic: Licensure Issues

36. Which action could jeopardize an ambulatory care nurse's licensure?

A) Maintaining certification in specialty areas

B) Failing to document patient care accurately

C) Following institutional protocols

D) Completing continuing education requirements

Topic: Incompetency and Informed Consent

37. How should a nurse handle a situation where a patient is deemed incompetent?

A) Proceed with care without consent

B) Seek consent from the patient's legal guardian or representative

C) Rely on verbal consent from family members

D) Delay all care until competency is restored

Topic: Legal and Ethical Issues

38. What is an ethical violation in ambulatory care?

A) Protecting patient confidentiality

B) Discriminating against a patient based on their socioeconomic status

C) Advocating for patient needs

D) Reporting unsafe practices

Topic: Skills and Knowledge

39. What knowledge area is critical for ambulatory care nurses managing diabetes?

A) Understanding surgical interventions

B) Teaching self-management strategies, including insulin use

C) Specializing only in emergency care

D) Ignoring patient dietary habits

Topic: Leadership and Management

40. What leadership approach encourages teamwork in ambulatory care?

A) Autocratic leadership

B) Collaborative and participatory leadership

C) Avoiding decision-making

D) Delegating all tasks without oversight

Section 4: The Systems

Topic: Scheduling Patients

41. What scheduling approach improves efficiency in ambulatory care?

A) Randomized patient appointments

B) Grouping patients with similar care needs together

C) Scheduling all patients at the same time

D) Avoiding follow-ups

Topic: Environmental Safety Issues

42. What is a critical action to ensure patient safety in the ambulatory care setting?

A) Ignoring clutter in patient areas

B) Conducting regular inspections of equipment and facilities

C) Prioritizing aesthetics over functionality

D) Avoiding maintenance schedules

Topic: Conflict Resolution

43. What is an effective strategy for resolving conflicts in the healthcare team?

A) Ignoring the conflict until it resolves on its own

B) Encouraging open communication between conflicting parties

C) Allowing conflicts to escalate to senior management immediately

D) Assigning blame to one party

Topic: Delegation of Duties

44. Which task should not be delegated to unlicensed assistive personnel (UAP)?

A) Assisting with ambulation

B) Collecting vital signs

C) Educating patients on medication side effects

D) Helping with activities of daily living

Topic: Managed Care Plans

45. What is a primary benefit of managed care plans for patients?

A) Restricting access to services

B) Coordinating comprehensive, cost-effective care

C) Avoiding preventative services

D) Increasing healthcare costs

Section 5: The Education

Topic: Health Promotion and Health Education

46. What is the focus of primary prevention in health promotion?

A) Early disease detection

B) Preventing the onset of disease through education and immunization

C) Rehabilitation after illness

D) Managing chronic diseases

Topic: Social Cognitive Theory

47. How does the concept of self-efficacy apply in Social Cognitive Theory?

A) Encouraging patients to depend on others

B) Empowering patients to believe in their ability to manage their health

C) Focusing only on external motivators

D) Avoiding patient feedback

Topic: Community Health

48. What is an example of a nurse's role in community health?

A) Providing health screenings at local events

B) Focusing solely on in-clinic care

C) Limiting services to insured individuals

D) Avoiding collaboration with public health organizations

Topic: Cultural Diversity

49. How can nurses demonstrate cultural competence in care delivery?

A) Assuming all patients have the same cultural practices

B) Asking patients about their cultural preferences and incorporating them into care plans

C) Avoiding discussions about cultural differences

D) Ignoring cultural beliefs to ensure standardized care

Topic: Primary, Secondary, and Tertiary Health Prevention

50. Which is an example of tertiary prevention in ambulatory care?

A) Administering vaccines to children

B) Providing education on healthy eating

C) Offering rehabilitation services to post-stroke patients

D) Conducting health fairs for early detection

Section 1: The Clinical Practice

Topic: Focal Points

51. What is an essential focal point in the management of patients with chronic illnesses in ambulatory care?

A) Emergency interventions

B) Consistent monitoring and patient education

C) Referral to inpatient care

D) Immediate surgical intervention

Topic: Patient Advocate

52. How can a nurse advocate for a patient experiencing difficulty accessing medication?

A) Ignore the patient's concerns

B) Direct them to alternative insurance options or assistance programs

C) Recommend they pay out of pocket

D) Suggest they stop the medication

Topic: Proper Triage

53. In ambulatory care, what should a nurse assess first during triage?

A) Patient demographics

B) Severity of symptoms and vital signs

C) Insurance information

D) Previous medical history

Topic: Qualifications

54. What certification can enhance an ambulatory care nurse's expertise in managing diabetes care?

A) Pediatric nursing certification

B) Certified Diabetes Care and Education Specialist (CDCES)

C) Advanced Trauma Life Support (ATLS)

D) Psychiatric nursing certification

Topic: Care Management

55. What is a key principle of patient-centered care management in ambulatory settings?

A) Prioritizing provider convenience

B) Customizing care plans to align with patient preferences and goals

C) Minimizing patient involvement in decision-making

D) Using the same care plan for all patients

Section 2: The Communication

Topic: Telehealth Nursing Skills

56. How should a nurse handle poor audio quality during a telehealth consultation?

A) End the consultation immediately

B) Switch to a secure alternative communication method

C) Continue without addressing the issue

D) Rely solely on written instructions

Topic: Documentation

57. What is the primary reason for documenting patient education in ambulatory care?

A) To meet insurance requirements

B) To provide a legal record of care and enhance continuity

C) To fulfill organizational policies

D) To reduce time spent with patients

Topic: Cultural Competence

58. Which practice demonstrates cultural competence when providing dietary advice?

A) Suggesting the same diet plan to all patients

B) Considering the patient's cultural food preferences and restrictions

C) Recommending only Western-style diets

D) Avoiding discussions about dietary habits

Topic: Service Recovery Process

59. How should a nurse respond to a patient complaint about long wait times?

A) Dismiss the complaint

B) Apologize sincerely and offer an explanation

C) Redirect the patient to another department

D) Ignore the issue

Topic: Informed Consent

60. What action should a nurse take if a patient expresses uncertainty about a procedure after signing the consent form?

A) Proceed with the procedure

B) Reassure the patient and clarify their concerns

C) Ignore the patient's uncertainty

D) Request the provider to force the decision

Section 3: The Professional Issues

Topic: Licensure Issues

61. What is a critical requirement for renewing a nursing license?

A) Completing continuing education requirements

B) Submitting only a renewal fee

C) Practicing without formal verification

D) Avoiding disciplinary action

Topic: Incompetency and Informed Consent

62. How should a nurse respond if a patient lacks the mental capacity to consent to treatment?

A) Ignore the issue and proceed with treatment

B) Involve the patient's legally authorized representative

C) Ask a colleague to make the decision

D) Avoid providing care

Topic: Legal and Ethical Issues

63. What action breaches patient confidentiality?

A) Sharing patient information with unauthorized individuals

B) Discussing patient cases with authorized care team members

C) Securing medical records in an electronic health system

D) Reporting unsafe practices to the authorities

Topic: Skills and Knowledge

64. Which knowledge area is essential for telehealth practice?

A) Advanced surgical skills

B) Proficiency in remote assessment tools

C) Knowledge of inpatient workflows

D) Focus on emergency-only care

Topic: Leadership and Management

65. What leadership style is most effective in promoting staff development?

A) Transformational leadership

B) Autocratic leadership

C) Passive leadership

D) Micromanagement

Section 4: The Systems

Topic: Scheduling Patients

66. How can nurses optimize scheduling for patients with multiple chronic conditions?

A) Avoid grouping appointments

B) Schedule comprehensive, multidisciplinary appointments

C) Limit appointment durations

D) Focus only on urgent cases

Topic: Environmental Safety Issues

67. What is a nurse's responsibility in ensuring environmental safety?

A) Reporting hazards immediately

B) Relying on maintenance staff only

C) Ignoring minor safety concerns

D) Avoiding interaction with the safety team

Topic: Conflict Resolution

68. What is a key skill for resolving conflict in patient care teams?

A) Active listening

B) Avoiding confrontation

C) Assigning blame

D) Ignoring disagreements

Topic: Delegation of Duties

69. What should a nurse consider before delegating a task?

A) The skill level of the person being delegated to

B) Whether the task is inconvenient for the nurse

C) Only the task's urgency

D) Avoiding task delegation

Topic: Managed Care Plans

70. How do managed care plans benefit healthcare providers?

A) By encouraging preventative care

B) By increasing patient load

C) By avoiding reimbursement processes

D) By limiting care to emergencies

Section 5: The Education

Topic: Health Promotion and Health Education

71. What is the nurse's role in health promotion for patients with hypertension?

A) Advising lifestyle modifications and routine screenings

B) Ignoring dietary concerns

C) Focusing solely on medication adherence

D) Suggesting no changes

Topic: Social Cognitive Theory

72. What strategy supports self-efficacy in patients managing obesity?

A) Providing achievable goals and positive reinforcement

B) Encouraging unrealistic goals

C) Avoiding discussions about weight

D) Focusing solely on group interventions

Topic: Community Health

73. How can nurses address public health challenges in underserved communities?

A) Partner with local organizations for outreach programs

B) Avoid community engagement

C) Focus solely on in-clinic care

D) Provide services only to insured patients

Topic: Cultural Diversity

74. How should nurses approach cultural diversity in health education?

A) Use culturally relevant examples and materials

B) Avoid addressing cultural differences

C) Ignore patient feedback on cultural preferences

D) Use a standard approach for all patients

Topic: Primary, Secondary, and Tertiary Health Prevention

75. What is an example of secondary prevention in ambulatory care?

A) Conducting annual mammograms for early detection

B) Teaching exercise routines

C) Administering post-operative physical therapy

D) Promoting vaccination programs

Section 1: The Clinical Practice

Topic: Focal Points

76. What is a primary responsibility of ambulatory care nurses in managing patient health?

A) Addressing acute illnesses only

B) Encouraging preventative care and health maintenance

C) Limiting interactions to follow-up visits

D) Avoiding long-term care coordination

Topic: Patient Advocate

77. How can an ambulatory care nurse effectively advocate for a patient with a new diagnosis?

A) Referring them to online resources only

B) Ensuring they have access to educational and community support resources

C) Avoiding discussions about the condition

D) Recommending they seek information on their own

Topic: Proper Triage

78. What is the primary goal of triage in ambulatory care?

A) Determining insurance coverage before care

B) Prioritizing care based on patient acuity

C) Offering identical care timelines to all patients

D) Delaying care until a physician is available

Topic: Qualifications

79. What additional qualification may benefit an ambulatory care nurse working with geriatric patients?

A) Pediatric advanced life support certification

B) Gerontological Nursing Certification (RN-BC)

C) Critical care nursing certification

D) Surgical nursing specialization

Topic: Care Management

80. What is a critical element of care management in ambulatory care?

A) Developing individualized care plans based on patient goals and conditions

B) Focusing only on acute care needs

C) Avoiding collaboration with other professionals

D) Using a one-size-fits-all care approach

Section 2: The Communication

Topic: Telehealth Nursing Skills

81. What should a nurse assess before initiating a telehealth session?

A) The patient's ability to travel

B) The patient's access to necessary technology

C) The patient's insurance provider

D) The time zone differences

Topic: Documentation

82. What is the best practice for documenting changes in a patient's treatment plan?

A) Including detailed reasons for changes in the medical record

B) Summarizing changes without details

C) Documenting only significant changes

D) Relying on verbal updates

Topic: Cultural Competence

83. How can a nurse demonstrate cultural competence when interacting with patients?

A) Assuming cultural preferences based on stereotypes

B) Asking patients about their beliefs and preferences

C) Avoiding discussions about culture

D) Using the same approach for all patients

Topic: Service Recovery Process

84. What is a proactive step in the service recovery process?

A) Waiting for the patient to file a formal complaint

B) Addressing patient concerns immediately

C) Ignoring minor complaints

D) Delegating all issues to management

Topic: Informed Consent

85. What must a nurse do to ensure informed consent?

A) Confirm that the patient understands all risks and benefits of the procedure

B) Assume the patient understands the procedure after a brief explanation

C) Avoid discussing alternatives

D) Focus solely on verbal communication

Section 3: The Professional Issues

Topic: Licensure Issues

86. How can nurses avoid licensure-related issues?

A) Meeting all continuing education requirements and maintaining ethical practices

B) Avoiding advanced certifications

C) Practicing without documentation

D) Limiting their professional development

Topic: Incompetency and Informed Consent

87. How should a nurse handle a situation where a patient's competency is questionable?

A) Request the patient sign the consent form immediately

B) Involve the patient's legal guardian or representative for decision-making

C) Avoid providing treatment

D) Proceed without consent

Topic: Legal and Ethical Issues

88. What is an example of an ethical violation in ambulatory care?

A) Breaching patient confidentiality

B) Collaborating with other professionals

C) Reporting unsafe practices

D) Educating patients about their treatment

Topic: Skills and Knowledge

89. Which skill is essential for ambulatory care nurses conducting patient education?

A) Strong communication and teaching skills

B) Proficiency in emergency medicine

C) Advanced surgical knowledge

D) Limited involvement in care planning

Topic: Leadership and Management

90. What leadership behavior builds trust within a nursing team?

A) Transparent communication and consistency

B) Micromanaging tasks

C) Avoiding team feedback

D) Delegating without providing support

Section 4: The Systems

Topic: Scheduling Patients

91. How can a nurse minimize patient wait times during scheduling?

A) Stagger appointments based on complexity and anticipated duration

B) Schedule multiple patients at the same time

C) Avoid asking about patient needs

D) Limit available appointment slots

Topic: Environmental Safety Issues

92. What is a key action to prevent falls in the clinic?

A) Keeping patient areas clear of clutter and spills

B) Ignoring safety concerns

C) Avoiding regular safety checks

D) Focusing only on staff safety

Topic: Conflict Resolution

93. What approach is effective in de-escalating workplace conflicts?

A) Active listening and collaborative problem-solving

B) Ignoring the issue until it resolves itself

C) Assigning blame

D) Avoiding involvement

Topic: Delegation of Duties

94. What task is appropriate to delegate to a certified nursing assistant (CNA)?

A) Assisting patients with hygiene and mobility needs

B) Administering intravenous medications

C) Educating patients on medication usage

D) Developing care plans

Topic: Managed Care Plans

95. What is a goal of managed care plans?

A) Improving care coordination and reducing healthcare costs

B) Limiting patient options for care

C) Avoiding preventative services

D) Increasing healthcare expenditures

Section 5: The Education

Topic: Health Promotion and Health Education

96. How can nurses support smoking cessation efforts?

A) Offering tailored education and resources to quit smoking

B) Ignoring the patient's smoking habit

C) Recommending no intervention

D) Avoiding the topic to save time

Topic: Social Cognitive Theory

97. What role does modeling play in Social Cognitive Theory?

A) Demonstrating healthy behaviors for patients to emulate

B) Avoiding examples in education

C) Focusing only on verbal instructions

D) Relying solely on group education

Topic: Community Health

98. What is a nurse's role in improving health outcomes in low-income communities?

A) Providing education on nutrition and preventative care

B) Limiting services based on income

C) Avoiding public health initiatives

D) Focusing solely on hospital-based care

Topic: Cultural Diversity

99. How can a nurse ensure inclusivity in patient care?

A) Using culturally relevant communication styles and materials

B) Assuming cultural preferences without discussion

C) Applying identical care approaches to all patients

D) Ignoring cultural beliefs

Topic: Primary, Secondary, and Tertiary Health Prevention

100. What is an example of primary prevention in ambulatory care?

A) Providing vaccinations to children and adults

B) Conducting screenings for hypertension
C) Offering rehabilitation for stroke patients
D) Managing post-operative recovery

6.2 Answer Sheet - Practice Test 1

1. Answer: B) Preventative care
Explanation: Ambulatory care nurses focus on preventative care to reduce complications, improve patient outcomes, and decrease the need for emergency interventions in chronic disease management.

2. Answer: B) Ensuring patient autonomy and informed decision-making
Explanation: Nurses act as advocates by supporting patient rights, ensuring their preferences are considered, and empowering them to make informed healthcare decisions.

3. Answer: B) Identifying the urgency of a patient's condition
Explanation: Proper triage involves quickly assessing a patient's condition and prioritizing care based on clinical urgency to ensure timely intervention.

4. Answer: C) Proficiency in chronic disease management and patient education
Explanation: Ambulatory care nurses must excel in managing chronic conditions and educating patients to ensure effective self-management.

5. Answer: C) Integrating multidisciplinary care plans
Explanation: Effective care management involves coordinating with various healthcare professionals to provide comprehensive care tailored to the patient's needs.

6. Answer: B) Proficient use of verbal and visual cues

Explanation: Telehealth requires nurses to rely on verbal and visual cues to assess the patient's condition accurately since physical examination isn't possible.

7. Answer: C) To provide a clear, comprehensive patient care record

Explanation: Proper documentation ensures continuity of care, enhances communication among the care team, and meets legal and regulatory requirements.

8. Answer: C) Recognizing one's own cultural biases

Explanation: Self-awareness is critical to understanding and respecting the cultural beliefs and practices of patients, which improves communication and care quality.

9. Answer: C) Acknowledging the patient's concerns and resolving issues promptly

Explanation: Effective service recovery involves actively listening to patient complaints, addressing issues quickly, and ensuring patient satisfaction.

10. Answer: B) The patient understands the risks, benefits, and alternatives of the procedure

Explanation: Informed consent requires ensuring that the patient has all necessary information to make an educated decision about their care.

11. Answer: B) An active RN license in good standing

Explanation: Maintaining an active RN license is fundamental for practicing as an ambulatory care nurse and meeting legal requirements.

12. Answer: A) When the patient is under duress

Explanation: Informed consent must be given voluntarily without coercion or pressure; otherwise, it is not valid.

13. Answer: C) Autonomy

Explanation: Respecting patient autonomy includes maintaining confidentiality and ensuring their personal information is protected.

14. Answer: B) Advanced critical thinking and decision-making

Explanation: Ambulatory care nurses must utilize critical thinking and make sound decisions to address the diverse and often complex needs of their patients.

15. Answer: C) Effective communication and team collaboration

Explanation: Strong communication and teamwork foster a productive environment, ensuring the team delivers high-quality care.

16. Answer: B) Prioritizing based on clinical urgency

Explanation: Scheduling patients based on clinical needs ensures timely care and better outcomes, especially for high-risk patients.

17. Answer: B) Conducting regular safety checks for patient areas

Explanation: Nurses must proactively ensure that the physical environment is safe for both patients and staff to prevent accidents and hazards.

18. Answer: B) Identifying the root cause of the disagreement

Explanation: Understanding the underlying issue helps address conflicts constructively and facilitates resolution.

19. Answer: B) Administration of routine medications

Explanation: Delegation must align with the scope of practice of the healthcare provider. Routine medication administration falls within the LPN's scope.

20. Answer: B) Reducing overall healthcare costs while maintaining quality

Explanation: Managed care focuses on cost-effectiveness and quality improvement by coordinating services and emphasizing prevention.

21. Answer: B) Empowering patients to adopt healthy lifestyle behaviors

Explanation: Health promotion involves encouraging patients to make informed choices that lead to better overall health outcomes.

22. Answer: B) By modeling healthy behaviors and encouraging self-efficacy

Explanation: Social Cognitive Theory highlights the importance of role modeling and building confidence in patients to improve behavior change.

23. Answer: B) Addressing social determinants of health

Explanation: Community health emphasizes understanding and mitigating factors like socioeconomic status and environment that affect health outcomes.

24. Answer: B) Learning about and respecting each patient's cultural background

Explanation: Recognizing and respecting cultural diversity leads to personalized care and improves patient trust and outcomes.

25. Answer: B) Conducting regular health screenings

Explanation: Secondary prevention focuses on early detection and intervention to halt the progression of diseases.

26. Answer: B) Prevention and chronic disease management

Explanation: Ambulatory care nursing emphasizes wellness by promoting preventative measures and supporting patients in managing chronic conditions.

27. Answer: B) Ensuring the patient fully understands their treatment options

Explanation: Advocacy involves empowering patients with knowledge to make informed decisions that align with their values and preferences.

28. Answer: B) To determine the order of care based on medical urgency
Explanation: Triage helps prioritize care to manage resources effectively and address patients' needs based on clinical severity.

29. Answer: A) Certification in telehealth nursing
Explanation: Telehealth certification ensures nurses are equipped to handle virtual consultations and manage remote care effectively.

30. Answer: C) Care management plans tailored to individual needs
Explanation: Individualized care management plans help patients navigate chronic conditions and ensure continuity of care.

31. Answer: A) Ensuring a secure and private communication platform
Explanation: Secure platforms protect patient confidentiality and are crucial for effective telehealth communication.

32. Answer: B) It allows immediate updates for continuity of care
Explanation: Real-time documentation ensures accuracy, reduces errors, and enhances communication across the healthcare team.

33. Answer: B) Use professional medical interpreters
Explanation: Professional interpreters ensure accurate communication and reduce the risk of misinterpretation, promoting culturally competent care.

34. Answer: D) Ensuring the problem doesn't happen again
Explanation: Service recovery is complete when systemic improvements are implemented to prevent recurring issues.

35. Answer: B) When the nurse confirms patient comprehension of the procedure
Explanation: Informed consent requires that the patient fully understands the risks, benefits, and alternatives before agreeing to the procedure.

36. Answer: B) Failing to document patient care accurately

Explanation: Poor documentation can lead to legal and ethical consequences, jeopardizing licensure.

37. Answer: B) Seek consent from the patient's legal guardian or representative

Explanation: When a patient is incompetent, legal representatives must provide consent to ensure ethical care.

38. Answer: B) Discriminating against a patient based on their socioeconomic status

Explanation: Ethical practice requires equitable treatment for all patients, regardless of their background.

39. Answer: B) Teaching self-management strategies, including insulin use

Explanation: Educating patients on managing their diabetes is vital for effective long-term care.

40. Answer: B) Collaborative and participatory leadership

Explanation: Collaborative leadership fosters trust and teamwork, ensuring better patient outcomes.

41. Answer: B) Grouping patients with similar care needs together

Explanation: Efficient scheduling optimizes staff time and reduces patient wait times.

42. Answer: B) Conducting regular inspections of equipment and facilities

Explanation: Regular inspections identify and mitigate potential hazards, ensuring a safe environment for patients and staff.

43. Answer: B) Encouraging open communication between conflicting parties

Explanation: Open communication helps clarify misunderstandings and fosters mutual understanding to resolve conflicts amicably.

44. Answer: C) Educating patients on medication side effects

Explanation: Patient education requires the expertise of licensed professionals to ensure accurate and safe information delivery.

45. Answer: B) Coordinating comprehensive, cost-effective care

Explanation: Managed care plans aim to provide coordinated care that balances quality with cost efficiency.

46. Answer: B) Preventing the onset of disease through education and immunization

Explanation: Primary prevention focuses on proactive measures to avoid the development of diseases.

47. Answer: B) Empowering patients to believe in their ability to manage their health

Explanation: Self-efficacy is central to Social Cognitive Theory, emphasizing the patient's confidence in their ability to succeed.

48. Answer: A) Providing health screenings at local events

Explanation: Nurses play a vital role in promoting public health through community outreach and preventative services.

49. Answer: B) Asking patients about their cultural preferences and incorporating them into care plans

Explanation: Cultural competence involves understanding and respecting diverse cultural practices to provide patient-centered care.

50. Answer: C) Offering rehabilitation services to post-stroke patients
Explanation: Tertiary prevention focuses on minimizing the impact of an established disease through rehabilitation and therapy.

51. Answer: B) Consistent monitoring and patient education
Explanation: Continuous monitoring and education empower patients to manage their chronic illnesses effectively, reducing complications.

52. Answer: B) Direct them to alternative insurance options or assistance programs
Explanation: Advocacy includes connecting patients to resources that address barriers to accessing necessary treatments.

53. Answer: B) Severity of symptoms and vital signs
Explanation: Evaluating symptoms and vital signs helps prioritize care based on the patient's immediate needs.

54. Answer: B) Certified Diabetes Care and Education Specialist (CDCES)
Explanation: The CDCES credential demonstrates expertise in diabetes care and education, crucial for managing this common condition in ambulatory care.

55. Answer: B) Customizing care plans to align with patient preferences and goals
Explanation: Patient-centered care ensures that treatment plans are tailored to individual needs and values, promoting better outcomes.

56. Answer: B) Switch to a secure alternative communication method
Explanation: Maintaining clear communication is essential, and secure alternatives ensure the quality and confidentiality of telehealth services.

57. Answer: B) To provide a legal record of care and enhance continuity
Explanation: Documenting education ensures that care is traceable and supports consistent follow-up.

58. Answer: B) Considering the patient's cultural food preferences and restrictions
Explanation: Incorporating cultural dietary habits makes advice more practical and acceptable for the patient.

59. Answer: B) Apologize sincerely and offer an explanation
Explanation: Acknowledging the complaint and explaining steps to address it demonstrates commitment to improving service.

60. Answer: B) Reassure the patient and clarify their concerns
Explanation: Informed consent is an ongoing process, and addressing patient concerns ensures they remain confident in their decision.

61. Answer: A) Completing continuing education requirements
Explanation: Continuing education ensures nurses maintain current knowledge and skills, meeting state board requirements.

62. Answer: B) Involve the patient's legally authorized representative
Explanation: Consent must be obtained from a representative if the patient is unable to provide it.

63. Answer: A) Sharing patient information with unauthorized individuals
Explanation: Confidentiality is a fundamental ethical and legal responsibility in nursing.

64. Answer: B) Proficiency in remote assessment tools
Explanation: Remote tools are vital for accurate patient evaluation in telehealth settings.

65. Answer: A) Transformational leadership
Explanation: Transformational leaders inspire and empower team members to achieve their full potential.

66. Answer: B) Schedule comprehensive, multidisciplinary appointments
Explanation: Coordinating care across specialties reduces the need for multiple visits and enhances patient outcomes.

67. Answer: A) Reporting hazards immediately
Explanation: Prompt reporting prevents accidents and ensures a safe environment for all.

68. Answer: A) Active listening
Explanation: Active listening helps identify and address the root cause of conflicts.

69. Answer: A) The skill level of the person being delegated to
Explanation: Delegation must align with the individual's competence and scope of practice.

70. Answer: A) By encouraging preventative care
Explanation: Managed care plans incentivize preventive care to improve outcomes and reduce costs.

71. Answer: A) Advising lifestyle modifications and routine screenings
Explanation: Educating patients on diet, exercise, and regular check-ups is key to managing hypertension.

72. Answer: A) Providing achievable goals and positive reinforcement
Explanation: Setting realistic goals builds confidence and fosters behavior change.

73. Answer: A) Partner with local organizations for outreach programs
Explanation: Collaboration expands access to care and resources, addressing social determinants of health.

74. Answer: A) Use culturally relevant examples and materials
Explanation: Tailoring education to cultural contexts increases engagement and effectiveness.

75. Answer: A) Conducting annual mammograms for early detection
Explanation: Secondary prevention focuses on early detection and treatment to prevent disease progression.

76. Answer: B) Encouraging preventative care and health maintenance
Explanation: Preventative care and health maintenance reduce the risk of complications and improve long-term patient outcomes.

77. Answer: B) Ensuring they have access to educational and community support resources
Explanation: Advocacy includes connecting patients to resources that help them navigate their diagnosis and access support.

78. Answer: B) Prioritizing care based on patient acuity
Explanation: Effective triage ensures that patients with the most urgent needs receive timely care.

79. Answer: B) Gerontological Nursing Certification (RN-BC)
Explanation: Specializing in gerontological nursing equips nurses to address the unique needs of older adults.

80. Answer: A) Developing individualized care plans based on patient goals and conditions
Explanation: Tailoring care plans ensures that they address specific patient needs and preferences, promoting better outcomes.

81. Answer: B) The patient's access to necessary technology
Explanation: Ensuring that patients have the required tools for a telehealth session is essential for effective communication and care delivery.

82. Answer: A) Including detailed reasons for changes in the medical record

Explanation: Comprehensive documentation ensures clarity and continuity of care.

83. Answer: B) Asking patients about their beliefs and preferences

Explanation: Open communication ensures that care aligns with the patient's cultural values and needs.

84. Answer: B) Addressing patient concerns immediately

Explanation: Timely responses build trust and improve patient satisfaction.

85. Answer: A) Confirm that the patient understands all risks and benefits of the procedure

Explanation: Informed consent requires the patient to have a full understanding of the procedure, its risks, benefits, and alternatives.

86. Answer: A) Meeting all continuing education requirements and maintaining ethical practices

Explanation: Compliance with licensure requirements ensures nurses remain qualified and practice within legal boundaries.

87. Answer: B) Involve the patient's legal guardian or representative for decision-making

Explanation: Patients unable to provide informed consent require a legally authorized representative to make decisions on their behalf.

88. Answer: A) Breaching patient confidentiality

Explanation: Confidentiality is a cornerstone of ethical nursing practice, and breaches can harm patient trust and violate legal obligations.

89. Answer: A) Strong communication and teaching skills

Explanation: Effective education requires the ability to convey information clearly and engage patients in their care.

90. Answer: A) Transparent communication and consistency

Explanation: Trust is fostered through clear communication and fair, consistent behavior.

91. Answer: A) Stagger appointments based on complexity and anticipated duration

Explanation: Scheduling adjustments ensure that care flows efficiently and minimizes delays.

92. Answer: A) Keeping patient areas clear of clutter and spills

Explanation: A safe environment reduces the risk of falls and ensures patient well-being.

93. Answer: A) Active listening and collaborative problem-solving

Explanation: Addressing conflicts through communication fosters resolution and teamwork.

94. Answer: A) Assisting patients with hygiene and mobility needs

Explanation: Tasks within the CNA's scope include basic patient care activities.

95. Answer: A) Improving care coordination and reducing healthcare costs

Explanation: Managed care focuses on efficiency and cost-effectiveness while maintaining quality.

96. Answer: A) Offering tailored education and resources to quit smoking

Explanation: Smoking cessation programs improve health outcomes and reduce risks associated with tobacco use.

97. Answer: A) Demonstrating healthy behaviors for patients to emulate
Explanation: Patients are more likely to adopt behaviors they observe in trusted role models.

98. Answer: A) Providing education on nutrition and preventative care
Explanation: Education empowers individuals to make healthier choices and access available resources.

99. Answer: A) Using culturally relevant communication styles and materials
Explanation: Inclusivity involves respecting and adapting to each patient's cultural context.

100. Answer: A) Providing vaccinations to children and adults
Explanation: Primary prevention focuses on measures to prevent the onset of disease.

7.1 FULL-LENGTH PRACTICE TEST 2

Section 1: The Clinical Practice

Topic: Focal Points

101. What is the nurse's primary focus when managing patients with multiple chronic conditions?

A) Providing emergency care

B) Ensuring effective coordination of care across providers

C) Limiting the number of follow-up visits

D) Prioritizing acute care needs only

Topic: Patient Advocate

102. How can a nurse advocate for a patient facing language barriers?

A) Relying on family members for interpretation

B) Using professional interpreters to facilitate communication

C) Limiting patient education until barriers are resolved

D) Avoiding discussions on complex topics

Topic: Proper Triage

103. Which patient would be prioritized during triage in an ambulatory care setting?

A) A patient with stable chronic back pain

B) A patient reporting chest pain and shortness of breath

C) A patient requesting routine medication refill

D) A patient with a mild skin rash

Topic: Qualifications

104. Which skill is crucial for ambulatory care nurses to enhance patient engagement?

A) Surgical assistance

B) Motivational interviewing

C) Inpatient monitoring

D) Advanced diagnostic testing

Topic: Care Management

105. How can a nurse ensure continuity of care during patient transitions?

A) Providing a detailed care summary to the patient and other providers

B) Limiting care discussions to in-office visits

C) Avoiding communication with external providers

D) Delegating all responsibilities to the patient

Section 2: The Communication

Topic: Telehealth Nursing Skills

106. What is an essential consideration when providing telehealth services?

A) Assessing and adapting to the patient's comfort with technology

B) Ignoring technical difficulties

C) Focusing only on verbal communication

D) Avoiding the use of visual aids

Topic: Documentation

107. How should a nurse document a patient's reported symptoms?

A) Using the patient's exact words in quotation marks

B) Paraphrasing symptoms based on the nurse's interpretation

C) Avoiding detailed symptom descriptions

D) Documenting only severe symptoms

Topic: Cultural Competence

108. What is a culturally competent way to address dietary needs?

A) Suggesting dietary plans aligned with the patient's cultural preferences

B) Providing generic diet recommendations

C) Avoiding dietary discussions

D) Assuming cultural preferences based on appearance

Topic: Service Recovery Process

109. What is a nurse's priority when managing a service complaint?

A) Listening to the patient's concern without interrupting

B) Explaining why the complaint isn't valid

C) Ignoring the issue

D) Referring the patient to management immediately

Topic: Informed Consent

110. When is informed consent required in ambulatory care?

A) Before initiating any invasive procedure

B) Only for procedures involving anesthesia

C) After completing the procedure

D) Only when requested by the patient

Section 3: The Professional Issues

Topic: Licensure Issues

111. What is an essential step in maintaining an active nursing license?

A) Completing all required continuing education hours

B) Practicing without renewal

C) Skipping professional development

D) Avoiding license renewal fees

Topic: Incompetency and Informed Consent

112. How should a nurse respond if a patient shows signs of confusion during a consent discussion?

A) Reassess the patient's understanding and involve family or a legal guardian if needed

B) Proceed with obtaining consent

C) Ignore the confusion

D) Cancel the procedure entirely

Topic: Legal and Ethical Issues

113. What action demonstrates adherence to ethical standards in nursing?

A) Protecting patient confidentiality at all times

B) Discussing patient information in public areas

C) Ignoring institutional policies

D) Avoiding ethical dilemmas

Topic: Skills and Knowledge

114. What knowledge area is essential for ambulatory care nurses managing medication reconciliation?

A) Familiarity with common drug interactions and patient-specific factors

B) Expertise in surgical interventions

C) Knowledge of inpatient workflows

D) Focusing only on generic prescriptions

Topic: Leadership and Management

115. What is an effective leadership approach to managing team conflicts?

A) Facilitating open communication and collaboration

B) Avoiding involvement in conflicts

C) Assigning blame to team members

D) Ignoring team dynamics

Section 4: The Systems

Topic: Scheduling Patients

116. How can a nurse improve scheduling efficiency in a busy clinic?

A) Streamlining appointments based on patient complexity and staff availability

B) Overbooking appointment slots

C) Avoiding follow-up scheduling

D) Ignoring patient time constraints

Topic: Environmental Safety Issues

117. What is a critical step to ensuring safety during equipment use?

A) Conducting regular maintenance checks

B) Assuming equipment is functional without inspection

C) Delaying maintenance requests

D) Using outdated equipment

Topic: Conflict Resolution

118. How can nurses prevent conflicts in patient care teams?

A) Establishing clear communication and defined roles

B) Ignoring potential disagreements

C) Allowing team members to work without guidance

D) Focusing only on individual tasks

Topic: Delegation of Duties

119. What task should a nurse avoid delegating to unlicensed staff?

A) Monitoring and documenting patient vital signs

B) Educating patients on complex treatment regimens

C) Assisting patients with mobility

D) Collecting routine specimens

Topic: Managed Care Plans

120. What is a nurse's role in a managed care plan?

A) Coordinating care among multiple providers to improve patient outcomes

B) Limiting access to healthcare services

C) Ignoring preventative care measures

D) Focusing only on short-term treatments

Section 5: The Education

Topic: Health Promotion and Health Education

121. What is the focus of tertiary prevention in health education?

A) Helping patients manage chronic diseases and prevent complications

B) Administering vaccinations

C) Screening for early disease detection

D) Encouraging smoking cessation

Topic: Social Cognitive Theory

122. How can a nurse apply Social Cognitive Theory in patient education?

A) Modeling positive behaviors and providing reinforcement for changes

B) Limiting patient feedback

C) Focusing only on theoretical explanations

D) Ignoring patient motivation

Topic: Community Health

123. How can a nurse promote health equity in underserved communities?

A) Advocating for access to resources and preventative care

B) Focusing only on insured patients

C) Avoiding involvement in public health initiatives

D) Providing only acute care services

Topic: Cultural Diversity

124. What is an essential practice for nurses working with culturally diverse populations?

A) Adapting communication styles to align with the patient's cultural norms

B) Using the same approach for all patients

C) Avoiding cultural discussions

D) Assuming cultural preferences

Topic: Primary, Secondary, and Tertiary Health Prevention

125. What is an example of secondary prevention in ambulatory care?

A) Performing annual blood pressure screenings

B) Administering childhood vaccinations

C) Providing cardiac rehabilitation

D) Educating patients on healthy diets

Section 1: The Clinical Practice

Topic: Focal Points

126. What is a key focus for ambulatory care nurses in managing acute exacerbations of chronic diseases?

A) Ensuring immediate hospitalization

B) Preventing complications through early intervention

C) Avoiding patient follow-up

D) Relying on emergency departments for care

Topic: Patient Advocate

127. How can a nurse advocate for a patient with limited access to care?

A) Refer the patient to community health programs and resources

B) Suggest the patient seek care in another city

C) Avoid addressing the access issue

D) Focus only on in-office care

Topic: Proper Triage

128. During triage, which factor should be assessed first?

A) The patient's financial status

B) The urgency of the patient's symptoms

C) The patient's preference for treatment location

D) The availability of the physician

Topic: Qualifications

129. What specialized training may benefit a nurse providing telehealth services?

A) Training in remote communication and technology use

B) Specialization in surgical procedures

C) Emergency medical technician (EMT) certification

D) Training in inpatient workflows

Topic: Care Management

130. What is a critical consideration in managing care for patients with multiple chronic conditions?

A) Coordinating interdisciplinary care plans

B) Focusing on a single condition at a time

C) Limiting care coordination to the primary provider

D) Avoiding the use of technology

Section 2: The Communication

Topic: Telehealth Nursing Skills

131. How should a nurse verify patient understanding during a telehealth session?

A) Request the patient to restate the care plan in their own words

B) Assume the patient understood the information

C) Provide a brief summary and end the session

D) Focus only on written instructions

Topic: Documentation

132. Why is documenting patient allergies essential in ambulatory care?

A) To reduce medication errors and adverse reactions

B) To meet legal requirements only

C) To avoid additional paperwork

D) To ensure consistency in insurance claims

Topic: Cultural Competence

133. What is an effective way for a nurse to learn about a patient's cultural preferences?

A) Asking open-ended questions about their beliefs and practices

B) Assuming the patient's culture based on appearance

C) Avoiding discussions about culture

D) Following standard protocols for all patients

Topic: Service Recovery Process

134. What is the first step in handling a service complaint effectively?

A) Apologizing and actively listening to the patient's concerns

B) Providing a detailed explanation without acknowledging the issue

C) Redirecting the complaint to another department

D) Ignoring the concern if it seems minor

Topic: Informed Consent

135. How should a nurse ensure informed consent is valid?

A) Verify that the patient comprehends the procedure and its implications

B) Focus solely on obtaining a signature

C) Skip explaining the risks of the procedure

D) Provide minimal information to avoid confusion

Section 3: The Professional Issues

Topic: Licensure Issues

136. What is a consequence of practicing nursing with an expired license?

A) Revocation of licensure and legal penalties

B) Automatic renewal upon request

C) Continuation of practice without issue

D) Avoiding patient care responsibilities

Topic: Incompetency and Informed Consent

137. What should a nurse do if a patient is declared legally incompetent?

A) Obtain consent from the patient's legal guardian or representative

B) Proceed with treatment without consent

C) Delay care indefinitely

D) Avoid contacting legal representatives

Topic: Legal and Ethical Issues

138. What is an example of a legal responsibility for nurses in ambulatory care?

A) Ensuring accurate documentation of patient care

B) Sharing patient information with unauthorized individuals

C) Skipping incident reports for minor issues

D) Providing care without patient consent

Topic: Skills and Knowledge

139. Which skill is essential for effective patient teaching in ambulatory care?

A) The ability to simplify complex medical information

B) Expertise in advanced diagnostic techniques

C) Proficiency in surgical procedures

D) Limiting interactions with patients

Topic: Leadership and Management

140. What leadership style is most effective in a team-based ambulatory care setting?

A) Collaborative leadership with active team involvement

B) Autocratic leadership with no team input

C) Passive leadership with minimal oversight

D) Avoidance of leadership responsibilities

Section 4: The Systems

Topic: Scheduling Patients

141. How can a nurse reduce scheduling conflicts in a busy practice?

A) Using an electronic scheduling system to streamline appointments

B) Avoiding appointment reminders

C) Limiting appointment slots arbitrarily

D) Overbooking to accommodate potential cancellations

Topic: Environmental Safety Issues

142. What is a nurse's responsibility in maintaining a safe environment?

A) Reporting and addressing potential hazards promptly

B) Ignoring minor safety issues

C) Leaving safety checks to other staff

D) Focusing only on patient care tasks

Topic: Conflict Resolution

143. What strategy helps de-escalate conflicts in patient care teams?

A) Encouraging open dialogue and mutual respect

B) Assigning blame to specific team members

C) Ignoring team concerns

D) Avoiding conflict resolution altogether

Topic: Delegation of Duties

144. Which task is appropriate for delegation to a licensed practical nurse (LPN)?

A) Administering routine medications

B) Performing initial patient assessments

C) Developing care plans

D) Educating patients on complex treatments

Topic: Managed Care Plans

145. What is the focus of managed care plans in ambulatory settings?

A) Enhancing preventative care and reducing costs

B) Limiting patient options for care

C) Avoiding follow-up visits

D) Increasing healthcare expenses

Section 5: The Education

Topic: Health Promotion and Health Education

146. What is a nurse's role in health promotion for patients with obesity?

A) Providing education on lifestyle modifications and physical activity

B) Ignoring the patient's weight concerns

C) Focusing only on medication therapy

D) Avoiding discussions about diet and exercise

Topic: Social Cognitive Theory

147. What strategy can nurses use to encourage behavior change using Social Cognitive Theory?

A) Setting achievable goals and offering consistent feedback

B) Focusing only on verbal instructions

C) Ignoring patient motivation

D) Relying solely on peer influence

Topic: Community Health

148. How can nurses address community health disparities?

A) Partnering with local organizations to provide health education and screenings

B) Limiting services to insured individuals

C) Focusing only on acute care

D) Avoiding collaboration with public health initiatives

Topic: Cultural Diversity

149. How can a nurse ensure cultural sensitivity when delivering patient education?

A) Adapting materials to align with the patient's cultural background

B) Using generic materials for all patients

C) Avoiding discussions about cultural beliefs

D) Assuming all patients share the same preferences

Topic: Primary, Secondary, and Tertiary Health Prevention

150. What is an example of tertiary prevention in ambulatory care?

A) Providing rehabilitation services for stroke recovery

B) Administering flu vaccines

C) Conducting regular blood pressure screenings

D) Educating about healthy eating habits

Section 1: The Clinical Practice

Topic: Focal Points

151. What is a critical focal point for nurses in ambulatory care when addressing mental health issues?

A) Immediate referral to inpatient care

B) Integrating mental health support with primary care services

C) Avoiding discussions on mental health topics

D) Focusing only on physical health

Topic: Patient Advocate

152. How does a nurse act as an advocate during a care plan discussion?

A) Ensuring the patient's preferences and goals are incorporated

B) Encouraging the provider to make all decisions

C) Limiting the patient's involvement in decision-making

D) Avoiding discussions about alternatives

Topic: Proper Triage

153. Which triage action is most appropriate for a patient presenting with severe abdominal pain?

A) Advising the patient to wait for a routine appointment

B) Escalating care immediately for evaluation

C) Scheduling the patient within a week

D) Reassuring the patient without further assessment

Topic: Qualifications

154. What qualification enhances a nurse's role in providing patient education on medications?

A) Certification in pharmacology or medication management

B) Specialization in emergency procedures

C) Advanced skills in surgical support

D) Knowledge limited to general nursing

Topic: Care Management

155. How can nurses promote effective care management for patients with diabetes?

A) Coordinating nutritional counseling and regular monitoring

B) Focusing only on medication adherence

C) Avoiding discussions about lifestyle changes

D) Limiting care to clinic visits

Section 2: The Communication

Topic: Telehealth Nursing Skills

156. How can nurses build rapport with patients during telehealth consultations?

A) Using empathetic communication and active listening

B) Focusing solely on technical details

C) Limiting personal interactions

D) Avoiding video consultations

Topic: Documentation

157. What should be included when documenting a patient's care plan?

A) Clear objectives, interventions, and expected outcomes

B) Personal opinions about the patient

C) Vague descriptions of the care process

D) Only short-term goals

Topic: Cultural Competence

158. What is a nurse's priority when caring for patients with diverse cultural beliefs?

A) Respecting and accommodating cultural practices

B) Ignoring cultural differences

C) Encouraging patients to adopt the nurse's preferences

D) Limiting communication about cultural topics

Topic: Service Recovery Process

159. What is the primary goal of the service recovery process?

A) Restoring patient trust and satisfaction

B) Avoiding acknowledgment of mistakes

C) Limiting patient feedback opportunities

D) Redirecting complaints to other departments

Topic: Informed Consent

160. What is a nurse's role in the informed consent process?

A) Ensuring the patient fully understands the procedure and alternatives

B) Obtaining a signature without explanation

C) Allowing only the provider to discuss consent

D) Avoiding detailed discussions

Section 3: The Professional Issues

Topic: Licensure Issues

161. What action demonstrates professional responsibility in maintaining licensure?

A) Completing continuing education requirements on time

B) Practicing without renewal

C) Avoiding professional development activities

D) Skipping license renewal fees

Topic: Incompetency and Informed Consent

162. How should a nurse handle a situation where a patient's competency is temporarily impaired?

A) Postpone non-urgent procedures and reassess competency later

B) Proceed without consent

C) Obtain consent from any family member available

D) Disregard the impairment

Topic: Legal and Ethical Issues

163. What is an ethical responsibility of nurses in ambulatory care?

A) Reporting unsafe practices to the appropriate authority

B) Ignoring minor patient safety concerns

C) Avoiding involvement in ethical dilemmas

D) Skipping incident reports

Topic: Skills and Knowledge

164. What skill is critical for managing patient transitions of care?

A) Effective communication with patients and other providers

B) Limiting communication to written records

C) Avoiding care coordination

D) Delegating all tasks to administrative staff

Topic: Leadership and Management

165. How can a nurse leader effectively promote team collaboration?

A) Encouraging open communication and shared decision-making

B) Avoiding team discussions

C) Delegating all tasks without guidance

D) Ignoring team input

Section 4: The Systems

Topic: Scheduling Patients

166. What strategy improves scheduling efficiency in high-volume clinics?

A) Implementing reminder systems to reduce no-shows

B) Overbooking slots

C) Ignoring patient preferences

D) Limiting appointment availability

Topic: Environmental Safety Issues

167. What is the nurse's role in maintaining safety in ambulatory care settings?

A) Identifying and mitigating hazards proactively

B) Waiting for others to report safety concerns

C) Ignoring minor risks

D) Avoiding involvement in safety protocols

Topic: Conflict Resolution

168. What is an essential step in resolving conflicts between team members?

A) Identifying the root cause of the conflict

B) Assigning blame without discussion

C) Avoiding involvement in conflicts

D) Limiting communication between team members

Topic: Delegation of Duties

169. What task should not be delegated to unlicensed assistive personnel (UAP)?

A) Assisting with activities of daily living

B) Performing patient education on disease management

C) Collecting routine specimens

D) Measuring vital signs

Topic: Managed Care Plans

170. What is a primary focus of managed care in ambulatory settings?

A) Providing cost-effective, preventative care services

B) Limiting patient access to care

C) Prioritizing acute interventions only

D) Avoiding care coordination

Section 5: The Education

Topic: Health Promotion and Health Education

171. What is an example of health promotion in ambulatory care?

A) Educating patients about smoking cessation programs

B) Providing acute care for infections

C) Administering post-surgical rehabilitation

D) Focusing solely on medication compliance

Topic: Social Cognitive Theory

172. How can nurses use Social Cognitive Theory to support patient adherence to treatment plans?

A) Demonstrating positive behaviors and providing encouragement

B) Limiting patient involvement in care

C) Focusing only on verbal instructions

D) Ignoring patient feedback

Topic: Community Health

173. What is a nurse's role in addressing public health challenges?

A) Advocating for access to preventative care and education

B) Limiting services to individual patients only

C) Avoiding participation in community health programs

D) Focusing solely on private care

Topic: Cultural Diversity

174. How can nurses respect cultural diversity in care plans?

A) Incorporating the patient's cultural values and beliefs into treatment

B) Using a standardized care plan for all patients

C) Ignoring cultural differences

D) Assuming all patients share similar values

Topic: Primary, Secondary, and Tertiary Health Prevention

175. What is an example of secondary prevention in ambulatory care?

A) Screening for colorectal cancer in at-risk patients

B) Educating patients on healthy eating

C) Administering flu vaccines

D) Providing cardiac rehabilitation

Section 1: The Clinical Practice

Topic: Focal Points

176. What is a key focus for ambulatory care nurses in managing preventative care?

A) Performing emergency interventions

B) Educating patients on lifestyle changes to reduce risks

C) Relying solely on medication management

D) Focusing only on acute care

Topic: Patient Advocate

177. How can a nurse act as an advocate for a patient needing specialist care?

A) Coordinating referrals and ensuring timely access to specialists

B) Leaving referral decisions entirely to the patient

C) Avoiding discussions about specialist care

D) Focusing only on primary care needs

Topic: Proper Triage

178. What is a nurse's first step when triaging a patient with symptoms of a stroke?

A) Escalating the case immediately for emergency care

B) Scheduling the patient for a routine visit

C) Advising the patient to monitor symptoms at home

D) Completing an extended history before taking action

Topic: Qualifications

179. What additional qualification enhances a nurse's ability to manage telehealth services?

A) Certification in virtual care or telehealth nursing

B) Training in surgical procedures

C) Pediatric nursing certification

D) Emergency response certification

Topic: Care Management

180. What is the nurse's role in care management for patients transitioning between providers?

A) Providing detailed care summaries to facilitate continuity

B) Limiting communication with new providers

C) Avoiding involvement in patient transitions

D) Relying solely on administrative staff for transitions

Section 2: The Communication

Topic: Telehealth Nursing Skills

181. How can a nurse address a patient's technical difficulties during a telehealth session?

A) Offering guidance on resolving issues or rescheduling if necessary

B) Ending the session without assistance

C) Ignoring the issue and continuing the consultation

D) Suggesting the patient switch to in-person care permanently

Topic: Documentation

182. Why is it important to document patient refusals of treatment?

A) To provide a legal record and support informed decision-making

B) To avoid further discussions with the patient

C) To ensure the patient cannot change their mind later

D) To document the provider's frustration

Topic: Cultural Competence

183. How can a nurse provide culturally sensitive care during end-of-life discussions?

A) Respecting the patient's cultural beliefs and practices regarding death

B) Avoiding discussions about end-of-life care

C) Assuming all patients have the same preferences

D) Recommending standard protocols regardless of culture

Topic: Service Recovery Process

184. What is a nurse's role in resolving service complaints effectively?

A) Listening to the patient's concerns and providing solutions promptly

B) Dismissing minor complaints

C) Referring all complaints to management without discussion

D) Ignoring the patient's feedback

Topic: Informed Consent

185. How can a nurse confirm a patient's understanding of informed consent?

A) Asking the patient to explain the procedure, risks, and benefits in their own words

B) Providing only written information

C) Assuming the patient understands without verification

D) Focusing only on the provider's explanation

Section 3: The Professional Issues

Topic: Licensure Issues

186. How can a nurse ensure compliance with licensure requirements?

A) Keeping accurate records of completed continuing education credits

B) Skipping professional development activities

C) Avoiding license renewals

D) Practicing without verification

Topic: Incompetency and Informed Consent

187. What action should a nurse take if a patient lacks the capacity to make decisions?

A) Involve a legal guardian or healthcare proxy to provide consent

B) Proceed without consent to save time

C) Delay all care indefinitely

D) Avoid contacting legal representatives

Topic: Legal and Ethical Issues

188. What is an example of a legal violation in ambulatory care?

A) Failing to maintain patient confidentiality

B) Reporting unsafe practices

C) Following evidence-based guidelines

D) Documenting care accurately

Topic: Skills and Knowledge

189. What skill is critical for nurses managing patients with multiple medications?

A) Proficiency in medication reconciliation

B) Expertise in surgical procedures

C) Knowledge of only over-the-counter drugs

D) Avoiding discussions about prescriptions

Topic: Leadership and Management

190. What leadership approach fosters a positive workplace culture?

A) Transparent communication and recognition of team efforts

B) Avoiding team discussions entirely

C) Micromanaging all team activities

D) Limiting collaboration

Section 4: The Systems

Topic: Scheduling Patients

191. How can a nurse reduce patient wait times in a busy practice?

A) Using automated appointment reminders and optimizing time slots

B) Scheduling multiple patients at the same time

C) Ignoring patient preferences

D) Overbooking routinely

Topic: Environmental Safety Issues

192. What is a nurse's priority in maintaining a safe environment?

A) Conducting regular safety inspections and addressing hazards promptly

B) Waiting for patients to report safety concerns

C) Ignoring minor risks

D) Delegating safety responsibilities to non-clinical staff

Topic: Conflict Resolution

193. What is an essential component of conflict resolution in patient care teams?

A) Active listening and mutual respect

B) Assigning blame without discussion

C) Ignoring the conflict until it resolves itself

D) Avoiding communication entirely

Topic: Delegation of Duties

194. What task can appropriately be delegated to unlicensed assistive personnel (UAP)?

A) Assisting with patient hygiene and mobility

B) Educating patients about complex disease management

C) Administering intravenous medications

D) Developing comprehensive care plans

Topic: Managed Care Plans

195. How do managed care plans promote efficiency in healthcare?

A) Coordinating services and emphasizing preventative care

B) Focusing only on emergency treatments

C) Reducing access to necessary services

D) Avoiding follow-ups

Section 5: The Education

Topic: Health Promotion and Health Education

196. What is the nurse's role in promoting health for patients at risk of cardiovascular disease?

A) Educating about diet, exercise, and routine health screenings

B) Ignoring lifestyle factors

C) Recommending only medication therapy

D) Limiting discussions about prevention

Topic: Social Cognitive Theory

197. How can nurses apply Social Cognitive Theory in promoting healthy behaviors?

A) Encouraging goal setting and providing positive reinforcement

B) Avoiding discussions about behavior change

C) Focusing solely on group education

D) Ignoring individual patient needs

Topic: Community Health

198. How can nurses address health disparities in underserved populations?

A) Advocating for access to care and resources

B) Limiting services to insured individuals

C) Avoiding community health initiatives

D) Focusing only on acute care

Topic: Cultural Diversity

199. How can a nurse demonstrate cultural competence when planning care?

A) Tailoring care to align with the patient's cultural beliefs and preferences

B) Using a standardized approach for all patients

C) Ignoring cultural considerations

D) Assuming all patients share similar values

Topic: Primary, Secondary, and Tertiary Health Prevention

200. What is an example of primary prevention in ambulatory care?

A) Administering childhood immunizations

B) Conducting cancer screenings

C) Providing post-operative rehabilitation

D) Educating patients about managing existing conditions

7.2 Answer Sheet - Practice Test 2

101. Answer: B) Ensuring effective coordination of care across providers
Explanation: Effective coordination reduces fragmentation in care and improves outcomes for patients with chronic conditions.

102. Answer: B) Using professional interpreters to facilitate communication
Explanation: Professional interpreters ensure accurate communication, empowering patients to make informed decisions.

103. Answer: B) A patient reporting chest pain and shortness of breath
Explanation: Symptoms such as chest pain and shortness of breath suggest a potential medical emergency and require immediate attention.

104. Answer: B) Motivational interviewing
Explanation: Motivational interviewing encourages patients to take an active role in their care, fostering engagement and behavior change.

105. Answer: A) Providing a detailed care summary to the patient and other providers
Explanation: Clear communication during transitions prevents gaps in care and ensures better outcomes.

106. Answer: A) Assessing and adapting to the patient's comfort with technology

Explanation: Adapting to the patient's technological proficiency ensures effective communication and delivery of care.

107. Answer: A) Using the patient's exact words in quotation marks
Explanation: Accurate documentation preserves the patient's voice and provides a clear record of their concerns.

108. Answer: A) Suggesting dietary plans aligned with the patient's cultural preferences
Explanation: Culturally tailored recommendations are more likely to be followed and effective.

109. Answer: A) Listening to the patient's concern without interrupting
Explanation: Active listening demonstrates empathy and is the first step in resolving patient dissatisfaction.

110. Answer: A) Before initiating any invasive procedure
Explanation: Informed consent is a legal and ethical requirement prior to invasive treatments or procedures.

111. Answer: A) Completing all required continuing education hours
Explanation: Continuing education ensures nurses stay up-to-date with best practices and licensure requirements.

112. Answer: A) Reassess the patient's understanding and involve family or a legal guardian if needed
Explanation: Ensuring the patient's comprehension is vital to upholding ethical and legal standards of consent.

113. Answer: A) Protecting patient confidentiality at all times
Explanation: Confidentiality is a core ethical principle in nursing and ensures patient trust and privacy.

114. Answer: A) Familiarity with common drug interactions and patient-specific factors

Explanation: Accurate medication reconciliation prevents errors and ensures patient safety.

115. Answer: A) Facilitating open communication and collaboration

Explanation: Leaders who promote dialogue and teamwork help resolve conflicts and strengthen team cohesion.

116. Answer: A) Streamlining appointments based on patient complexity and staff availability

Explanation: Efficient scheduling balances staff resources and patient needs, reducing delays and enhancing care delivery.

117. Answer: A) Conducting regular maintenance checks

Explanation: Routine maintenance ensures equipment reliability and prevents safety hazards.

118. Answer: A) Establishing clear communication and defined roles

Explanation: Preventing conflict involves clear expectations and open dialogue among team members.

119. Answer: B) Educating patients on complex treatment regimens

Explanation: Patient education on complex care requires a nurse's expertise and licensure.

120. Answer: A) Coordinating care among multiple providers to improve patient outcomes

Explanation: Nurses play a critical role in ensuring that care is well-coordinated and patient-centered.

121. Answer: A) Helping patients manage chronic diseases and prevent complications

Explanation: Tertiary prevention aims to improve quality of life by reducing disease-related complications.

122. Answer: A) Modeling positive behaviors and providing reinforcement for changes

Explanation: Patients are more likely to adopt behaviors when they see them modeled effectively and receive positive reinforcement.

123. Answer: A) Advocating for access to resources and preventative care

Explanation: Nurses play a vital role in addressing health disparities by connecting communities to resources.

124. Answer: A) Adapting communication styles to align with the patient's cultural norms

Explanation: Tailored communication ensures understanding and builds trust with diverse populations.

125. Answer: A) Performing annual blood pressure screenings

Explanation: Secondary prevention focuses on early detection and intervention to halt disease progression.

126. Answer: B) Preventing complications through early intervention

Explanation: Ambulatory care nurses aim to manage acute exacerbations effectively to prevent the need for hospitalization and complications.

127. Answer: A) Refer the patient to community health programs and resources

Explanation: Connecting patients to accessible programs helps address barriers to care and ensures continuity.

128. Answer: B) The urgency of the patient's symptoms

Explanation: Determining the severity of symptoms ensures that the most critical cases receive prompt attention.

129. Answer: A) Training in remote communication and technology use
Explanation: Specialized training in telehealth equips nurses to effectively deliver care in virtual settings.

130. Answer: A) Coordinating interdisciplinary care plans
Explanation: Collaboration across disciplines ensures comprehensive care that addresses all aspects of the patient's health.

131. Answer: A) Request the patient to restate the care plan in their own words
Explanation: Asking the patient to explain their understanding ensures clarity and reinforces the care plan.

132. Answer: A) To reduce medication errors and adverse reactions
Explanation: Accurate documentation of allergies prevents errors and ensures patient safety.

133. Answer: A) Asking open-ended questions about their beliefs and practices
Explanation: Engaging patients in discussions about their culture helps tailor care to their preferences.

134. Answer: A) Apologizing and actively listening to the patient's concerns
Explanation: Addressing concerns with empathy and attentiveness demonstrates commitment to quality care.

135. Answer: A) Verify that the patient comprehends the procedure and its implications
Explanation: Informed consent requires the patient to fully understand the procedure, risks, benefits, and alternatives.

136. Answer: A) Revocation of licensure and legal penalties
Explanation: Practicing without a valid license violates legal and professional standards, leading to serious consequences.

137. Answer: A) Obtain consent from the patient's legal guardian or representative
Explanation: Legally incompetent patients require authorized representatives to make decisions on their behalf.

138. Answer: A) Ensuring accurate documentation of patient care
Explanation: Proper documentation ensures legal compliance and continuity of care.

139. Answer: A) The ability to simplify complex medical information
Explanation: Breaking down medical terms into understandable language helps patients engage in their care.

140. Answer: A) Collaborative leadership with active team involvement
Explanation: Collaboration promotes trust, enhances teamwork, and improves patient care outcomes.

141. Answer: A) Using an electronic scheduling system to streamline appointments
Explanation: Technology improves scheduling efficiency and reduces errors.

142. Answer: A) Reporting and addressing potential hazards promptly
Explanation: Identifying and addressing hazards ensures a safe environment for patients and staff.

143. Answer: A) Encouraging open dialogue and mutual respect
Explanation: Communication and respect are key to resolving conflicts and maintaining a positive work environment.

144. Answer: A) Administering routine medications

Explanation: LPNs can administer medications within their scope of practice, supporting the care team.

145. Answer: A) Enhancing preventative care and reducing costs

Explanation: Managed care emphasizes prevention and cost-effectiveness to improve patient outcomes.

146. Answer: A) Providing education on lifestyle modifications and physical activity

Explanation: Educating patients about diet and exercise helps them adopt healthier lifestyles.

147. Answer: A) Setting achievable goals and offering consistent feedback

Explanation: Realistic goals and feedback build confidence and encourage sustainable behavior change.

148. Answer: A) Partnering with local organizations to provide health education and screenings

Explanation: Partnerships enhance access to care and resources in underserved communities.

149. Answer: A) Adapting materials to align with the patient's cultural background

Explanation: Tailored education respects cultural values and improves understanding.

150. Answer: A) Providing rehabilitation services for stroke recovery

Explanation: Tertiary prevention focuses on improving quality of life and reducing disability after a disease has occurred.

151. Answer: B) Integrating mental health support with primary care services

Explanation: Addressing mental health within the primary care setting ensures holistic patient care and improved access to mental health resources.

152. Answer: A) Ensuring the patient's preferences and goals are incorporated
Explanation: Advocacy involves empowering patients to actively participate in their care planning process.

153. Answer: B) Escalating care immediately for evaluation
Explanation: Severe abdominal pain can indicate urgent conditions requiring prompt medical attention.

154. Answer: A) Certification in pharmacology or medication management
Explanation: Advanced certification ensures expertise in educating patients about medication usage, side effects, and safety.

155. Answer: A) Coordinating nutritional counseling and regular monitoring
Explanation: Comprehensive care management addresses multiple facets of diabetes control, including diet, exercise, and medication.

156. Answer: A) Using empathetic communication and active listening
Explanation: Rapport-building fosters trust and ensures effective communication in telehealth settings.

157. Answer: A) Clear objectives, interventions, and expected outcomes
Explanation: Detailed documentation supports continuity of care and ensures all team members are informed.

158. Answer: A) Respecting and accommodating cultural practices
Explanation: Culturally competent care promotes patient satisfaction and adherence to treatment.

159. Answer: A) Restoring patient trust and satisfaction

Explanation: Service recovery aims to address concerns and rebuild positive relationships with patients.

160. Answer: A) Ensuring the patient fully understands the procedure and alternatives

Explanation: Nurses play a vital role in clarifying information and confirming patient comprehension.

161. Answer: A) Completing continuing education requirements on time

Explanation: Continuing education ensures competence and compliance with licensure standards.

162. Answer: A) Postpone non-urgent procedures and reassess competency later

Explanation: Temporary impairments may resolve, allowing the patient to make informed decisions.

163. Answer: A) Reporting unsafe practices to the appropriate authority

Explanation: Nurses are ethically obligated to advocate for patient safety and report risks.

164. Answer: A) Effective communication with patients and other providers

Explanation: Clear communication ensures continuity and minimizes errors during care transitions.

165. Answer: A) Encouraging open communication and shared decision-making

Explanation: Collaboration fosters teamwork, enhances problem-solving, and improves patient care.

166. Answer: A) Implementing reminder systems to reduce no-shows
Explanation: Reminder systems help optimize schedules and reduce missed appointments.

167. Answer: A) Identifying and mitigating hazards proactively
Explanation: Proactive measures prevent accidents and promote a safe environment.

168. Answer: A) Identifying the root cause of the conflict
Explanation: Addressing the root cause allows for effective resolution and improved teamwork.

169. Answer: B) Performing patient education on disease management
Explanation: Education requires licensed professionals with specialized knowledge.

170. Answer: A) Providing cost-effective, preventative care services
Explanation: Managed care emphasizes prevention to improve outcomes and reduce costs.

171. Answer: A) Educating patients about smoking cessation programs
Explanation: Health promotion focuses on preventative measures to improve long-term well-being.

172. Answer: A) Demonstrating positive behaviors and providing encouragement
Explanation: Role modeling and reinforcement increase the likelihood of adherence.

173. Answer: A) Advocating for access to preventative care and education
Explanation: Nurses contribute to public health by improving access and promoting prevention.

174. Answer: A) Incorporating the patient's cultural values and beliefs into treatment
Explanation: Tailored care plans improve patient trust and adherence.

175. Answer: A) Screening for colorectal cancer in at-risk patients
Explanation: Secondary prevention aims to detect and treat diseases at an early stage.

176. Answer: B) Educating patients on lifestyle changes to reduce risks
Explanation: Preventative care involves educating patients about lifestyle modifications to prevent illnesses and promote health.

177. Answer: A) Coordinating referrals and ensuring timely access to specialists
Explanation: Advocacy includes facilitating access to specialists and ensuring smooth transitions between providers.

178. Answer: A) Escalating the case immediately for emergency care
Explanation: Stroke symptoms require urgent intervention to minimize long-term damage and improve outcomes.

179. Answer: A) Certification in virtual care or telehealth nursing
Explanation: Certification in telehealth prepares nurses to manage virtual care efficiently and effectively.

180. Answer: A) Providing detailed care summaries to facilitate continuity
Explanation: Comprehensive communication ensures smooth transitions and reduces the risk of errors.

181. Answer: A) Offering guidance on resolving issues or rescheduling if necessary

Explanation: Assisting patients with technical issues ensures they receive care without unnecessary delays.

182. Answer: A) To provide a legal record and support informed decision-making
Explanation: Documenting refusals protects both the patient and the provider while ensuring clarity in care.

183. Answer: A) Respecting the patient's cultural beliefs and practices regarding death
Explanation: Culturally sensitive care involves acknowledging and incorporating patients' values into their care.

184. Answer: A) Listening to the patient's concerns and providing solutions promptly
Explanation: Addressing complaints directly and empathetically builds trust and enhances patient satisfaction.

185. Answer: A) Asking the patient to explain the procedure, risks, and benefits in their own words
Explanation: Confirming understanding ensures the patient makes an informed decision about their care.

186. Answer: A) Keeping accurate records of completed continuing education credits
Explanation: Maintaining records ensures compliance and facilitates smooth licensure renewal.

187. Answer: A) Involve a legal guardian or healthcare proxy to provide consent
Explanation: Legally authorized representatives make decisions when patients cannot provide consent themselves.

188. Answer: A) Failing to maintain patient confidentiality

Explanation: Breaching confidentiality violates legal and ethical standards, undermining patient trust.

189. Answer: A) Proficiency in medication reconciliation

Explanation: Accurate reconciliation ensures medication safety and prevents harmful interactions.

190. Answer: A) Transparent communication and recognition of team efforts

Explanation: Effective leaders foster trust and motivation by encouraging open communication and teamwork.

191. Answer: A) Using automated appointment reminders and optimizing time slots

Explanation: Efficient scheduling reduces delays and improves the patient experience.

192. Answer: A) Conducting regular safety inspections and addressing hazards promptly

Explanation: Proactive safety measures prevent accidents and ensure patient well-being.

193. Answer: A) Active listening and mutual respect

Explanation: Effective conflict resolution involves understanding all perspectives and fostering collaboration.

194. Answer: A) Assisting with patient hygiene and mobility

Explanation: UAPs are trained for basic patient care activities within their scope of practice.

195. Answer: A) Coordinating services and emphasizing preventative care
Explanation: Managed care plans streamline care delivery and reduce costs through coordinated efforts.

196. Answer: A) Educating about diet, exercise, and routine health screenings
Explanation: Preventative education reduces the risk of developing cardiovascular diseases.

197. Answer: A) Encouraging goal setting and providing positive reinforcement
Explanation: Social Cognitive Theory emphasizes self-efficacy and reinforcement to support behavior change.

198. Answer: A) Advocating for access to care and resources
Explanation: Advocacy improves access to preventative and primary care for vulnerable populations.

199. Answer: A) Tailoring care to align with the patient's cultural beliefs and preferences
Explanation: Cultural competence ensures care is respectful and relevant to the patient's background.

200. Answer: A) Administering childhood immunizations
Explanation: Primary prevention focuses on preventing disease before it occurs.

TEST-TAKING STRATEGIES

Preparing for the **Ambulatory Care Nursing Exam** is just as much about mastering content as it is about developing effective test-taking strategies and managing test anxiety. This section provides proven techniques to help you approach exam day with confidence and perform at your best.

Test-Taking Strategies

1. Understand the Exam Format

- Familiarize yourself with the structure of the exam:
    - **150 questions** (125 scored, 25 pretest).
    - Multiple-choice format.
    - **3-hour time limit**.
- Practice with full-length tests to simulate the real exam experience.

2. Read Questions Carefully

- Take your time to thoroughly read the question and all answer options.
- Pay close attention to keywords like **"best," "most," "first," or "except"**

to understand what the question is asking.

- Look for qualifiers such as **always, never, sometimes**, which can alter the meaning of the question.

3. Eliminate Incorrect Answers

- Narrow down your choices by eliminating clearly incorrect answers.

- Focus on the remaining options and select the most logical choice based on the scenario.

4. Use Logic and Reasoning

- Rely on your nursing knowledge and critical thinking skills.

- Consider the **nursing process (Assessment, Diagnosis, Planning, Implementation, and Evaluation)** to guide your decision-making.

- Choose the option that aligns with patient-centered care and safety.

5. Manage Your Time

- Allocate your time wisely:

    - Spend about **1 minute per question**.

    - Flag challenging questions and return to them later if time allows.

- Avoid dwelling too long on a single question.

6. Look for Clues

- Some questions may provide context or clues that can help you answer correctly.
- Use the process of elimination to uncover hidden hints within the question.

7. Don't Overthink

- Avoid second-guessing yourself unless you realize a clear mistake.
- Often, your first instinct is the correct one.

8. Answer Every Question

- There is no penalty for guessing, so never leave a question unanswered.
- Use educated guesses when you're unsure.

Overcoming Test Anxiety

1. Be Prepared

- Confidence comes from thorough preparation.
- Use this guide to cover all exam topics and practice extensively with the included tests.

2. Develop a Study Routine

- Establish a consistent study schedule to avoid last-minute cramming.
- Use active learning techniques, such as summarizing information or

teaching it to others, to enhance retention.

3. Practice Relaxation Techniques

- Before and during the exam, try these methods to stay calm:

    - **Deep Breathing:** Inhale for 4 seconds, hold for 4 seconds, and exhale for 4 seconds.

    - **Progressive Muscle Relaxation:** Tense and relax each muscle group to release tension.

    - **Visualization:** Picture yourself confidently completing the exam.

4. Get Adequate Rest

- Aim for at least **7-8 hours of sleep** the night before the exam. Rested minds perform better.

5. Stay Positive

- Replace negative thoughts with affirmations:

    - "I am well-prepared for this exam."

    - "I can handle this challenge with confidence."

    - "I am capable and knowledgeable."

6. Stay Healthy

- Eat a balanced meal before the exam to maintain energy levels.

- Stay hydrated but avoid excessive caffeine, which can heighten anxiety.

7. Arrive Early

- Arrive at the testing center or log in to the online platform well before the scheduled time.

- Familiarize yourself with the environment to feel more at ease.

8. Focus on the Present

- Concentrate on one question at a time instead of worrying about the entire test.

- Use a calm, steady pace to maintain focus.

9. Accept What You Can't Control

- Some questions may seem difficult or confusing. Accept this as part of the exam process and focus on doing your best.

10. Reflect and Reset

- If you feel overwhelmed during the test:
  - Take a brief moment to pause and reset.
  - Use relaxation techniques to regain composure.

Tips for Exam Day

- **Bring Necessary Items:** Ensure you have your ID, admission ticket, and any allowed materials.

- **Dress Comfortably:** Wear layers to adjust to the testing environment.

- **Listen to Instructions:** Pay close attention to the proctor's guidelines to avoid misunderstandings.

Final Words of Encouragement

Test-taking anxiety is normal, but it doesn't define your capabilities. Trust in your preparation, focus on your strengths, and remind yourself of the hard work you've put in. With the strategies outlined in this guide, you're equipped to face the **Ambulatory Care Nursing Exam** with clarity and confidence.

Take a deep breath—you've got this!

ADDITIONAL RESOURCES

To complement this study guide, here is a curated list of online resources and academic materials that can further enhance your preparation for the **Ambulatory Care Nursing Exam**. These resources provide supplemental knowledge, practical insights, and additional practice to solidify your understanding of ambulatory care nursing concepts.

Recommended Online Resources

1. American Nurses Credentialing Center (ANCC)

- **Website:** www.nursingworld.org/ancc
- **Why Use It?:**
    - Provides the official blueprint for the Ambulatory Care Nursing Exam.
    - Offers guidelines, policies, and updates related to the certification process.
    - Includes valuable resources for continuing education.

2. Ambulatory Care Nursing Review Courses

- **Examples:**
  - **Nurse.com:** www.nurse.com
  - **MedEdPortal:** www.mededportal.org

- **Why Use It?:**
  - Access interactive courses and webinars designed specifically for ambulatory care nursing.
  - Gain insights from industry experts through video tutorials and case studies.

3. The American Academy of Ambulatory Care Nursing (AAACN)

- **Website:** www.aaacn.org

- **Why Use It?:**
  - Offers a variety of educational resources, position papers, and tools related to ambulatory care nursing.
  - Provides access to forums and discussion groups for networking with other nursing professionals.

4. Practice Test Platforms

- **Examples:**
  - **TestPrepReview:** www.testprepreview.com
  - **Kaplan Nursing:** www.kaptest.com

- **Why Use It?**:
    - Take additional practice tests to familiarize yourself with the exam format.
    - Receive detailed explanations to reinforce learning.

5. National Institutes of Health (NIH)

- **Website:** www.nih.gov
- **Why Use It?**:
    - Access free resources, research articles, and patient education materials relevant to ambulatory care.

6. Online Medical Journals

- **Examples:**
    - **PubMed:** www.pubmed.ncbi.nlm.nih.gov
    - **Journal of Ambulatory Care Management (JACM):** www.journals.lww.com
- **Why Use It?**:
    - Stay updated on the latest research and best practices in ambulatory care.

7. YouTube Channels

- **Examples:**

- **RegisteredNurseRN:** www.youtube.com
- **Simplenursing:** www.youtube.com

- **Why Use It?:**
  - Watch concise, visually engaging videos on key nursing topics and test-taking strategies.

Recommended Academic Materials

1. Ambulatory Care Nursing Review Questions

- **Book:** *Core Curriculum for Ambulatory Care Nursing (4th Edition)*
- **Publisher:** American Academy of Ambulatory Care Nursing (AAACN)
- **Why Use It?:**
  - Comprehensive review of ambulatory care concepts.
  - Includes practice questions and case scenarios.

2. Nursing Textbooks

- **Examples:**
  - *Nursing Care in Ambulatory Settings: Issues and Models of Care* by T.M. Powell
  - *Foundations of Nursing Practice: Essential Concepts* by Lois White

- **Why Use It?**:
  - Explains fundamental nursing principles in outpatient care.
  - Serves as a detailed reference for both students and practicing nurses.

3. Clinical Guidelines

- **Book:** *Clinical Guidelines for Advanced Practice Nursing: An Interdisciplinary Approach* by Rebekah Kaplan
- **Why Use It?**:
  - Provides evidence-based practices and detailed care models for ambulatory care settings.

4. Test Preparation Guides

- **Examples:**
  - *Mosby's Review Questions for the NCLEX-RN Exam (Ambulatory Care Edition)*
  - *Saunders Comprehensive Review for the NCLEX-RN® Exam* by Linda Anne Silvestri
- **Why Use It?**:
  - Offers practice questions aligned with nursing certification exams.
  - Includes rationales to improve understanding of complex topics.

5. Ethical and Legal Considerations

- **Book:** *Legal and Ethical Issues for Nurses* by Ginny Wacker Guido

- **Why Use It?**:

  - Focuses on legal and ethical challenges specific to nursing practice.

6. Pharmacology Resources

- **Book:** *Pharmacology Made Incredibly Easy!* by Lippincott

- **Why Use It?**:

  - Explains pharmacological principles in an accessible and engaging way, helping with medication management topics.

7. Health Promotion and Education

- **Book:** *Health Promotion Throughout the Lifespan* by Carole Edelman and Elizabeth Kudzma

- **Why Use It?**:

  - Detailed overview of health education strategies relevant to outpatient care.

How to Use These Resources

1. Start with the content review provided in this guide to establish a strong foundation.

2. Use online resources to deepen your understanding of specific topics or clarify doubts.

3. Practice extensively with academic materials and online practice tests to build confidence and test readiness.

4. Stay updated with the latest research and guidelines to align your knowledge with current practices.

By incorporating these **recommended online resources and academic materials** into your study routine, you can strengthen your preparation, expand your knowledge base, and ensure success on the **Ambulatory Care Nursing Exam 2024-2025**. Good luck!

FINAL WORDS

A MESSAGE OF ENCOURAGEMENT

Congratulations on taking the first step toward achieving your **Ambulatory Care Nursing Certification**! The decision to embark on this journey reflects your dedication, passion, and commitment to excellence in nursing. Preparing for this exam is not just about earning a credential—it's about deepening your knowledge, honing your skills, and affirming your ability to provide exceptional care to your patients.

The Path to Success

This journey may feel overwhelming at times, but remember that every moment spent studying, every concept mastered, and every practice question answered brings you one step closer to your goal. Progress, no matter how small, is still progress. Stay focused, trust the process, and believe in your ability to succeed.

Tips to Keep Moving Forward:

- **Remember Your Why:** Think about why you chose this path—whether it's to enhance patient outcomes, advance your career, or challenge yourself to grow. Let your motivation guide you through the challenging days.

- **Celebrate Small Wins:** Each topic you master and each practice test you complete is an accomplishment. Acknowledge your efforts and celebrate the progress you've made.

- **Stay Positive:** Positive thoughts lead to positive outcomes. Believe in your preparation, and know that you are equipped to tackle this exam with confidence.

You've Got This

The **Ambulatory Care Nursing Exam** is a challenge, but it's one you're ready to face. You've prepared with diligence and determination, and you now hold the tools to succeed. On exam day, take a deep breath, trust your knowledge, and approach each question with calm and clarity.

Remember These Final Tips:

- **Stay Confident:** Trust in your preparation. You've worked hard, and you are ready.

- **Stay Calm:** Use relaxation techniques to keep nerves in check. Focus on one question at a time.

- **Stay Focused:** The exam is an opportunity to showcase your knowledge and skills.

A Brighter Future Awaits

This certification is not just a milestone; it's a gateway to new opportunities, professional growth, and personal fulfillment. It signifies your expertise in ambulatory care and your unwavering dedication to improving the lives of patients.

You are making a difference—one patient, one moment, and one achievement at a time.

Words of Inspiration

A Final Thank You

Thank you for trusting this guide as part of your preparation journey. We hope it has empowered you, inspired you, and provided the tools you need to succeed. As you step into the next phase of your career, know that you have the strength, knowledge, and determination to achieve greatness.

Good luck on your exam—you've got this!

EXPLORE OUR RANGE OF STUDY GUIDES

At Test Treasure Publication, we understand that academic success requires more than just raw intelligence or tireless effort—it requires targeted preparation. That's why we offer an extensive range of study guides, meticulously designed to help you excel in various exams across the USA.

Our Offerings

- **Medical Exams:** Conquer the MCAT, USMLE, and more with our comprehensive study guides, complete with practice questions and diagnostic tests.

- **Law Exams:** Get a leg up on the LSAT and bar exams with our tailored resources, offering theoretical insights and practical exercises.

- **Business and Management Tests:** Ace the GMAT and other business exams with our incisive guides, equipped with real-world examples and scenarios.

- **Engineering & Technical Exams:** Prep for the FE, PE, and other technical exams with our specialized guides, which delve into both fundamentals and complexities.

- **High School Exams:** Be it the SAT, ACT, or AP tests, our high school range is designed to give you a competitive edge.

- **State-Specific Exams:** Tailored resources to help you with exams unique to specific states, whether it's teacher qualification exams or state civil service exams.

Why Choose Test Treasure Publication?

- **Comprehensive Coverage:** Each guide covers all essential topics in detail.

- **Quality Material:** Crafted by experts in each field.

- **Interactive Tools:** Flashcards, online quizzes, and downloadable resources to complement your study.

- **Customizable Learning:** Personalize your prep journey by focusing on areas where you need the most help.

- **Community Support:** Access to online forums where you can discuss concerns, seek guidance, and share success stories.

Contact Us

For inquiries about our study guides, or to provide feedback, please email us at support@testtreasure.com.

Order Now

Ready to elevate your preparation to the next level? Visit our website www.testtreasure.com to browse our complete range of study guides and make your purchase.